Beyond the Headlines: The Brutal Reality of Heatwaves and the Need for Action

Youssva

First Printing, 2024

Table of Contents

CHAPTER ONE: Introduction

In imagining more accessible futures, I am yearning for an elsewhere

– and perhaps an "elsewhen" – in which disability is understood otherwise:

as political, as valuable, as integral. (Kafer, 2013, p.3)

I have been a social worker in various capacities for two decades. Along with work that addressed social injustice in my community, I have spent many volunteer hours engaged in environmental research projects. In addition to completing degrees in both psychology and social work, I have taken several of interest university courses in environmental studies, biology, and geography. Remarkably, throughout my employment and studies across these subject areas, meaningful connections between these domains were rarely made. Having had these concurrent interests and experiences, I began to reflect on how certain aspects of my work, studies, and health were connected. Specifically, while studying and working to protect the most vulnerable in my community (from at-risk parents to injured songbirds), I was also living with the decline of my health through multiple chronic illnesses. As climate change began to affect the weather patterns where I lived, I suffered from heightened disease symptoms due to extreme heat, humidity, forest fires, and other weather events. Struggling with the cost of lifesaving equipment, such as air conditioners, air purifiers, and numerous medications, I wondered how other people with disabilities were faring with the worsening reality of climate change. Particularly, as a social worker and person with degenerative health conditions, I wondered how federal and provincial policies were representing and positioning the diverse needs of persons with disabilities through conditions that are amplified by a changing climate.

In my preliminary research, I noted that persons with disabilities suffer unequally when climate disasters occur. For example, I discovered that during tropical storms, wildfires, and hurricanes, persons with disabilities fare worse and are frequently abandoned. In the documentary *The Right to be Rescued*, writer and director Jordan Melograna (2015) shares stories of Americans with disabilities who were left behind in the aftermath of Hurricane Katrina. These findings are echoed in recent academic works, which are starting to make connections between changing weather patterns, natural disasters, and issues of social justice. Relatedly, Gaskin et al. (2017) found that the "systems designed to assist people in times of emergency, in particular, are often inaccessible to people with disability" (p. 811). This research is startling, yet not surprising. The reality is that climate change has the greatest impact on the world's poorest and most marginalized people, a significant proportion of whom are persons with disabilities (Baker, 2012; Gaskin et al., 2017; Wolbring, 2009).

As a thesis student in a Master of Social Work program that seeks to develop strong anti-oppressive research and social policy analysis, I was drawn to examine government initiatives related to climate change and human health. Specifically, I wondered how the Canadian Federal Government was planning for and including persons with disabilities in their climate action plans. While I recognize that people with disabilities are not homogenous, many face insurmountable challenges in their daily lives, which range from inaccessible communities to social exclusion and financial insecurities (Malhotra & Isitt, 2017; Rimmerman, 2013; Wolbring, 2009). Experientially, I have found that many of the challenges persons with disabilities face do not relate to disabled bodies and minds at all;

rather, they extend from barriers that exist deep within an ableist society. As such, I explore some of these systemic inequities and corporealities in the chapters that follow.

A Personal Connection

According to Canada's Changing Climate Report (Bush & Lemmen, 2019), global warming over the past century is both indisputable and, in large part, due to human activities. Canadian climate data suggests that Canada's warming is about twice the global rate, and the effects include extreme weather and rising sea levels. Alarmingly, the climate effects we are seeing now are the result of past and present emissions, and these impacts are projected to worsen in coming years. Along with these changes in temperature, fires, rainfall and storms, climate change causes a host of other effects including disrupting food systems and food security (Wheeler & von Braun, 2013). This stark reality carries compounding concerns, as marginalized populations, including persons with disabilities, tend to be the most food insecure in our communities.

Temperature records continue to be broken annually, and heat has become a serious threat to human life, causing mortality, health complications, and hospitalizations (Saito et al., 2018; Santamouris, 2019). From my research on heat related deaths, mortality rates begin to spike as the temperature exceeds 27 degrees Celsius. This reality hit close to home for me as someone with a condition that causes systemic dehydration. Since I feel debilitating effects from high summer humidity in tandem with extreme heat, I am intimately aware of how high humidity interferes with sweating, one of the body's cool down mechanisms. Frighteningly, absolute humidity, the measure of the actual moisture in the air, is the second most common marker for heat mortality in the United States (Shindell, et al., 2020). More worrisome is the finding that only 8% of 2.8 billion people living in the hottest countries of the world have access to air conditioners (International Energy Agency, 2018).

To this end, a troubling experience I had in 2018 best captures why I am particularly interested in this research topic. In July of 2018, I drove across Canada. Specifically, I left a sweltering, humid Nova Scotia and passed through Quebec on my way to the University of Victoria in British Columbia. During this particular week, a heatwave killed more than 90 people in Quebec alone, with public health officials noting that many who perished had underlying physical and/or mental health conditions (Fleming, et al., 2018). In fact, it was later speculated that the death toll from heat related illness was much higher than previously reported, yet many deaths were attributed to chronic and acute illnesses alone, without linking temperature or access to appropriate provisions. With temperatures surpassing 40 degrees Celsius with the humidex, I remember the staggering misery and exhaustion I felt when walking from my air-conditioned vehicle to the grocery store and then finally into a hotel. I recall my mounting anxiety coupled with ominous physical health symptoms, as the temperature gauge in the car read 42 degrees. The sun was unrelenting on the highway and I had to keep ice packs on my legs and head, even with the car air conditioning set to maximum. If I did not have access to a support person, cool air in the vehicle I was driving, and in the hotel room where I slept, I am sure my fate would have been a grave one. Even with air conditioning in my vehicle, I was not able to manage the heat-related symptoms. I had to make frequent stops for hydration and ice-cubes in order to bring down my body temperature, as there is was no escaping the blazing hot sun on Canada's highways.

Later that same summer, a state of emergency was declared in British Columbia as the province faced a catastrophic number of forest fires, resulting in record quantities of unhealthy air; this polluted air was both the cause and exacerbation of many illnesses (Fayerman & Mahichi, 2018). When the smoke blanketed Victoria, I visited at least five stores to find they were all sold out of air purifiers, with the exception of one store which had $649.00 (plus taxes) Dyson models still in stock. I wondered what this reality meant for those who were not mobile and could not access these stores or the funds needed for this protective equipment. I remember being wheezy, out of breath, and exhausted during my search through the smoky city and throughout the entire month that the wildfires raged. I began to question how adaptation, and the imperative to be adaptive to climate-related changes in government strategies, may be applied to persons with disabilities who already contend with multiple barriers and complexities. Through these experiences it became clear that those who are prepared, mobile, and have ample resources (air conditioners, air purifiers, support systems) are better situated in the face of climate change.

Another pivotal experience that prompted me to consider such intersections as disability and poverty in the face of climate change was a 2018 Mi'kmawgi Climate Justice gathering at a Friendship Centre in Halifax, Nova Scotia. At this event, I was seated at a roundtable discussion on intersectionality, hosted by Dalhousie professor, health and environmental racism researcher Dr. Ingrid Waldron. We spoke about what an intersectional approach to climate justice would look like and we heard from Mi'kmaq community members, environmental justice scholars, and local grassroots activists. Issues faced by Indigenous communities, those living in poverty, rural farmers, persons of colour, queer communities, persons with disabilities, and isolated people were shared in our group's discussion. This gathering in particular served as early fuel for my thesis project, as the issues I contend with here are apropos, emerging not only from scholarly works, but are also relevant among community organizations and grassroots activists. In Chapter Three, I further outline how attending these events and immersing myself in communities that are engaged in intersectional climate justice work is central to my research paradigm.

As mentioned, I am not alone in my concern for the most marginalized in this emerging field of climate change policies. Many scholars are starting to look at how intersections of poverty, gender, race, health, and class are leaving certain groups disproportionately vulnerable to climate threats. Notably, Weissbecker (2011) summarizes the reality that climate change will likely continue to expose and exacerbate already existing health, social, political, and economic inequities. Similarly, Perkins (2019) notes that gender connects with other types of vulnerabilities such as ethnicity, sexuality, and disability to increase climate related risks. Indeed, climate change is becoming a magnifier of vulnerabilities that already exist in our communities (Tschakert, 2007; Dankelman, 2010; Henly-Shepard, 2018).

Further, in the pursuit of social justice, social workers are now being called upon to play a role in climate justice and environmental issues because of our commitments to human rights, poverty, and health care (Cumby, 2016). In 2014, the Intergovernmental Panel on Climate Change (IPCC) cited increasing evidence that people living with disabilities, chronic health conditions, people living in poverty, and other marginalized groups are particularly vulnerable to cumulative adverse effects of climate change. Notably, these populations experience more displacement, morbidity and mortality as a result of climate change (IPCC, 2014). In this most recent IPCC synthesis report, the United Nations summarized findings that show climate change will continue to adversely affect those who are already marginalized socially, culturally, politically, economically, and institutionally. Coupled with my own experiences, many of my friends and colleagues who identify as having a disability share stories of worsening health due to weather events, compounded by struggles they already experience in society. As such, my interest in how health and disability showed up within Canadian climate change strategies was deepened.

I ground this study in the examination of six prominent Federal Government climate change documents that were suggested to me by Canada's Minister of Environment and Climate Change. Applying a set of critical research questions, some of them informed by my own experience of disability and climate change, I sought to uncover how health and disability were situated within these documents. The data selection process will be further described in my methodology chapter. Through a primarily inductive reflexive thematic analysis, I examine the ways in which health and disability are positioned within the climate change strategies. Having said this, and in keeping with researcher reflexivity, I am unable to separate my own critical disability politic from this research. Thus, through a series of reflective questions, I also bring a transparent element of deduction to this project.

In Chapter Two, I pull together diverse theorizations related to my research topic, synthesizing broad conversations happening around social justice within environmental and climate scholarship. I further situate and define notable terms used by the Canadian Federal Government in climate change discussions, such as *adaptation, resilience, and vulnerability*. In Chapter Three, I expand upon my conceptual framework and highlight my research design and methods. Here, I describe in detail the methods and steps of Braun and Clarke's reflexive thematic analysis that I have utilized for my careful reading of the data. In this chapter, I also articulate the value of poststructural, intersectional, critical, and feminist-disability inspired approaches as applied to social justice research. In Chapter Four, I present my findings collated through themes and subthemes while providing select excerpts and quotes from my data set. Following a detailed reflexive thematic analysis of the data, I speak to how ableism is constituted and perpetuated through climate change documents and the implications this has in the lives of persons with disabilities. In Chapter Five, my final chapter, I discuss how dominant narratives in the field of climate change coalesce with hegemonic notions of health and disability. I highlight taken-for-granted assumptions about bodies and minds in the data and how these beliefs are manifesting within the Canadian Federal Government climate change documents and broader society. I conclude by anchoring my findings within larger theoretical conversations and activism in social justice spheres. In sharing the material impacts of ableism I observe in climate change documents, I provide some alternatives to these narratives while offering my hopes for a future direction of anti-oppressive climate change strategies.

CHAPTER TWO: The Relevant Literature

In this chapter, I present scholarly works from across the various domains I broach in this study and, in the next chapter, I detail the methods used to analyze my data. Chapter Three, thus, builds on the theoretical underpinnings that I introduce below. My journey through the literature was winding and often arduous since it necessitated an exploration of emerging and distinct areas of scholarship. In order to bring rigour to my data analysis process, I acquainted myself with bodies of work spanning several fields of thought.

First, I needed to familiarize myself with key terms and concepts used in both government and scientific climate change discussions. Many of these concepts, such as *resilience* and *vulnerability*, have taken-for-granted meanings in climate change domains, while disciplines committed to social justice offer rich critiques of the same terms. For example, in social work, feminist disability studies, and critical disability studies, such concepts are widely criticized for failing to account for structural oppressions and latent understandings of resilience and vulnerability. As such, the diverse subjects I explored in my literature review were, at times, conflicting and vexing. Indeed, my process of finding relevant research and making sense of connections in the literature extended beyond what I have summarized in this review, since I have been wholly challenged to reimagine both disability justice and climate justice.

As I began to question how health and disability showed up in government climate change strategies, I discovered that very few studies look critically at where, why, and how disability appears in government climate change literature. For this reason, I ventured into such disciplines as climate science, climate justice, environmental studies, political geography, social adaptation, feminist disability studies, critical disability studies, and intersectionality. Therefore, the sections that follow synthesize these often historically disparate fields while further illustrating the connections between them.

Social Impacts of Climate Change

Scholarly research is beginning to emerge around the social impacts of climate change and, more specifically, how climate threats disproportionately impact marginalized communities, including those who live with disabilities (Alston, 2015). According to Wolbring and Leopatra (2012), natural disasters, floods, storms, and heatwaves affect persons with disabilities more gravely than those with able bodies and minds. Relatedly, Kosanic et al., (2019) note that persons with disabilities often have limited access to climate resources, services, and information, while at the same time, their health conditions may be exacerbated by infectious diseases, climate-related events, and disasters. Endorsed by the National Aeronautics and Space Administration (NASA), the recent assessment of climate change on human health in the United States conclude that climate change creates new human health challenges and exacerbates existing health conditions through changing weather patterns and climatic conditions (Climate Science Special Report, 2018).

Given that climate change has proven and projected negative effects on all people, there is an increasing number of studies looking at the social implications of environmental issues. For example, Kaijser and Kronsell (2013) claim that the impacts of climate change are mediated through social structures as well as economic, and cultural practices, thereby underscoring the need for social analyses around these issues. While it is evident that climate change disproportionately impacts persons with disabilities and other historically marginalized communities, there is sparse literature available on how these processes are unfolding and what social work can contribute to mitigating these disparities. In the article

Social Work, Climate Change and Global Cooperation, Alston (2015) asks social workers to consider some critical factors when engaging with climate change and its social implications. Specifically, social workers are called to "differentiate between the impacts of climate events and existing social inequalities" (Alston, 2015, p. 356). With this in mind, I have paid particular attention to the structural inequities that already set the stage for inequalities in climate change mitigation strategies.

Ableism

Ableism is a useful term to situate in this study since the disability literature makes clear that ableism is pervasive, and it is often bound to other mechanisms of domination and normalization (Alston, 2015; Nocella, 2017; Simpson, 2017). These oppressive processes deeply entrench the marginalization of disabled people in society. Disability activist Mia Mingus (2011) points out that ableism connects to all of our challenges as disabled people, since it is secured by notions of whose bodies are important, desired, and disposable. In her writing, Mingus (2011) helps to illustrate the corporeal oppression of disabled people, highlighting the insidious ways in which hegemonic notions of the body impact the well-being of persons with disabilities. The book *Disability Politics and Theory* (Withers, 2012) echoes Mingus' sentiment that the struggles of those deemed to have a disability are often the consequence of active marginalization. Similarly, Wolbring (2008) defines ableism as "a set of beliefs and practices that produce – based on abilities one exhibits or values – a particular understanding of oneself, one's body and one's relationship" (p. 252). Related to the widespread subjugation of persons with disabilities, Rauscher and McClintock (2006) note that ableism manifests when:

> Deeply rooted beliefs about health, productivity, beauty and the value of human life, perpetuated by the public and private media, combine to create an environment that is hostile to those whose abilities fall outside of the scope of what is currently defined as socially acceptable. (p. 198)

Indeed, ableism is connected to discrimination and cultural beliefs that uphold notions of healthy and *normal* in contrast to illness and disability.

Alison Kafer (2013) states that ableist assumptions about bodies in turn influence realities of access, affecting both disabled and non-disabled people. In the *Crip Manifesto for Health Rebels,* Kafer (2017) suggests that we understand disability as relational, appearing and arising in the relations between people, policies, beliefs, and structures that surround all of us. While there is a need to address disproportionate resources and increasing environmental threats, scholars such as Kafer also call us to address our tendency to see health and disability as depoliticized, ahistorical facts.

Like many of the concepts I contend with in this study, ableism is a contested term. In fact, Withers (2012) suggests that ableism is a misnomer in that it implies that we are oppressed because of ability when we actually experience oppression because of disability. Further, many critical disability theorists refuse to provide a definition or construction of what or who represents a disabled body (Tremain, 2005). Yet, for the purposes of this study, I believe it is helpful to provide a contextualized overview and categorization of disabilities. Rohrer (2005) offers a useful summary of common disability categories:

> There are differences in type of disability (in a reification of the mind/body split, disability is usually broken down as physical or intellectual), in impact (minor hearing loss versus paralysis), in onset (disability from birth/gradually becoming

> disabled/suddenly becoming disabled), in perceptibility (having a 'hidden disability' and 'passing' as non-disabled versus being unable to hide a disability), in variability (most disabilities change across time and space), and in prevalence (disabilities vary by sex, ethnicity, age, and environment). (p. 41)

Of course, these are broad categories and often do not take into account the multiple intersections and nuance of illness and disability. My personal experience with chronic illness and disease leads me to conceptualize disability as inherently mutable, deeply political, and certainly situation specific. I see disability as nuanced and fluid, with my own experience of disability changing from space to space, dependent upon place and the company I keep. Similarly, Withers (2012) points out that disability is always in *flux*, and we move in and out of the category of disabled depending on the context.

Within the self-identified disability communities of which I am a part, ableism is the term mostly widely accepted to theorize our ongoing experiences of marginalization. That being said, Shildrick (2009) argues that by using categories of disabled and non-disabled, we uphold the binaries and systems that perpetuate our exclusions. I agree with this sentiment, yet at this point in time and for the purposes of my study, contextualizing the experiences of persons with disabilities remains a worthy endeavour, at least until the abled ⇔ disabled binary is bridged. Consequently, I view ableism as both a concept and a verb, a term that nods to the ongoing processes of oppression that many people face. Since I am exploring the ways in which persons with disabilities are showing up in this new field of climate change, ableism remains a useful term to describe a set of discriminatory beliefs and practices.

Medical and Social Models of Disability

There are several distinct disability models found in the literature: the *medical model* of disability and the *social model* of disability are historically the most common, and most relevant to my politics and research. Seccombe (2006) summarizes the medical model through its aligning disability with illness and cure, a categorization based on the pathophysiology of disabilities and normalization of specific bodies. Similarly, Crow (1996) notes that this model holds that "a person's functional limitations (impairments) are the root *cause* of any disadvantages experienced and these disadvantages can therefore only be rectified by treatment or cure" (p. 208). Conversely, the social model of disability acknowledges that people with disabilities may experience various challenges, yet the primary focus is on the disabling effects of society, including environmental obstacles, discrimination and financial stressors (Seccombe, 2006). In addition, according to the World Health Organization (2010), the social model recognizes that accessibility is the problem not dis/ability itself; while further, disability has both a causal and consequential relationship with poverty.

While these are widely accepted definitions, I note that some researchers have critiqued the social model of disability, largely for its failure to recognize the multiplicity of experiences (Shakespeare & Watson, 2010; Thomas, 2007). I address some of these concerns in both the intersectionality section of this chapter and in the chapters that follow. Disability certainly is a contested subject, one that Kafer (2013) suggests requires our departure from a social model of 'disabled' and 'non-disabled' as self-evident binary categories. This being said, I continue to most closely align myself with the social model of disability, its politics and relational understandings of abled/disabled. Throughout my research journey, I contemplate these categories and binaries of disability, specifically questioning their contradictory and taken-for-granted natures.

As I previously pointed out, disability exists in relation to how we view the other, how we speak about persons with chronic health challenges, and how we relate to ourselves and others. Kafer (2013) highlights the sweeping assumptions of able-bodiedness and able-mindedness that pervade writings about nature and environment. Similarly, Simpson (2017) contends that ableism has given license to medicine and science researchers to commit transgressions in the name of normalcy and health. Related to this finding, the impetus for this study includes my curiosity about how able-bodied and able-minded norms, or 'ableism' may be informing climate policies.

Like other environmental and social policies, climate change strategies are not natural or neutral responses; climate change decisions and the conditions that make disabled people more vulnerable stem from pre-existing political beliefs, institutional inequities, and systems of colonization and oppression. Anna Kirkland (2010) argues that health (or the appearance of health) bestows status to some while taking it away from others. Indeed, health as an ideal or norm, has been used against people and populations, with good health being marker of status and power. In the article, *A Culture of Neglect: Climate Discourse and Disabled People*, Wolbring (2009) warns that ableism is expected to prevail in the era of climate change, where people who are less affected by climate change are unwilling to adequately accommodate those who are more affected. Likewise, Simpson (2017) notes that disability and perceptions of disability are still used to justify the oppression of marginalized communities. While ideally, I would not reproduce and recite the categorization and binaries used to describe experiences of disabilities, I believe their current and historical significance has a place in my study.

Situating Critiques of Ableism and Climate Change Policies

Disability, as articulated by Grue (2011), is often characterized by a distinct pattern of systemic discrimination, stigma, and oppression. That said, rare nods to disability in climate change discussions tend not to reside in a category of their own but classified under the umbrella of *vulnerable populations*. Interestingly, in the Yale lecture "Why Preserve the Life of the Other", philosopher Judith Butler (2016) contends that labelling some as vulnerable presumes a didactic relationship in which the others who are charged with protecting the vulnerable are seen as invulnerable, thus fortifying a paternalistic relationship. This altruistic other seems to exist in discussions pertaining to climate change and vulnerable populations, a governing body who presents as a depoliticized savior. I used this insight as a guidepost to help me reflect on how government ideologies influence both the climate change strategies and our corporealities as disabled people.

Thiesmeyer (2003) defines ideologies as social representations that are shared by groups to accomplish everyday practices such as communicating, further noting that deep layers of ableist ideology and power are concealed within political documents. Jonathan Metzl (2010) offers additional reflection, calling health part of the problem we need to address and arguing that our attention should be placed on the tendency to see health, illness, disease, and disability as depoliticized ahistorical facts of the mind and body. Metzl (2010) suggests that calls for social justice to merely redistribute resources while ignoring damaging ideologies is to miss part of the problem. Social justice that is conceptualized as merely the redistribution resources assumes health is a fixed entity that can be transported or transferred to one setting or another (Metzl, 2010). Relatedly, Clare (2017) argues that this "ideology of cure" (p.15) speaks to our values of what is normal and natural, even what can be restored to a better condition. That is, when we speak about cure, we must first perceive something, or someone, as damaged, as needing to return to a former or more superior body-mind state (Clare, 2017). Although the scope of my study does not permit me to deeply interrogate these pervasive ideals of normal and natural body-minds, I include reference to these in my literature review as they help to contextualize my framework and analysis. This being said, my research is aligned with the type of disability justice articulated by Nocella (2017), one that celebrates uniqueness, difference and interdependence, a politic that recognizes everyone has varying types of abilities and experiences of health.

Problematizing Adaptation, Vulnerability, and Climate Resilience

It is important to note that in climate change literature at large, adaptation is one of the most widely used concepts related to mitigation efforts. Considered one of the leading authorities on climate change worldwide, the Intergovernmental Panel on Climate Change (IPCC, 2018) defines adaptation as processes of adjustment to real or anticipated climate effects. In Canadian government climate policy documents, the term adaptation is used analogously. For example, in a Health Canada publication recommended to me by Canada's Minister of Environment and Climate Change, the authors define climate change as "Adjustment in natural or human systems in response to actual or expected effects of climate change and variability, which moderates harm or exploits beneficial opportunities" (Seguin, 2008). Similarly, on their website, in a section devoted to adapting to climate change, the Government of Canada (2019) defines adaptation as the adjustments we make to our behaviours, decisions, and activities before or after current or anticipated climate changes. Since my study focuses on government climate change strategies that are largely informed by IPCC reports, these definitions are particularly useful. I define and contextualize these concepts early in my literature review, as they help to set the stage for how I have approached and analyzed my data. At the same time, like many of the concepts I address in this study, adaptation to climate change is a directive that is extensively critiqued. One significant criticism hinges on the fact that adaptation has no end point and consists of ongoing adjustments to climate change (Barnett et al., 2015). These critics argue that adaptation is not actually a solution to climate change, rather it is a set of actions that require constant, mounting, and shifting burdens. Equally essential to this research, is the notion that identifying successful adaptation measures is more about fairness and equity and the inherent viability of a process, rather than one particular outcome (Barnett et al., 2015; Hurlimann et al., 2014; Stafford-Smith et al., 2011).

Barriers and Limits to Climate Change

The terms *barriers* and *limits* are often used interchangeably in the literature on climate change adaptation, with select studies pointing to their different meanings. Moser and Ekstrom (2010) summarize the distinction between the two concepts, stating that limits often refer to absolute thresholds in biological and ecological systems, whereas barriers are obstacles that refer to shifts in thinking, land uses, management, distribution of resources, and priorities. Yet, like many emerging terms and concepts included in this study, "the distinction between barriers and limits to adaptation is ambiguous" (Barnett, et al., 2015, p. 6).

Jones and Boyd (2011) have identified cognitive, normative, and institutional factors as distinct yet connected variables that contribute to social barriers to adaptation. Resource disparities and financial struggles are factors that emerge in most of the research related to challenges to adaptation; yet the Canadian government does not implicate government welfare systems in their discussions. Related to this point, in studies that have looked at barriers to climate change adaptation in Nepal, "the hegemonic dominance of political authority, and the channels through which aid/resources are allocated by the upper caste stratum, are identified as key barriers in responding to shock and stress" (Jones & Boyd, 2011, p. 1270). Further, Filho and Knieling (2013) point to contextual challenges with adaptation, suggesting that adaptive capacities vary from country-to-country depending on economics, government systems, social structure, culture, available technology, and specific environmental threats. While more recently, in *Overcoming the Limits to Adaptation,* scholars critique current climate projects for being primarily sector-focused (such as farming) and offering benefits only to particular groups (Filho & Nalau, 2017). It is clear that, while adaptation is front and centre in Canada's response to climate change, the literature suggests that the meanings associated with adaptation and its usefulness within and across communities need to be further examined. With respect to what works and what does not work in successful climate change adaptation approaches, Filho and Nalau (2017) share the following:

> The promotion and dissemination of good practice is one of the ways to convincingly show the diversity of the limits to adaptation and likewise the diversity of strategies to address these. There are plenty of lessons from the past showing what works and what does not. Left unattended however, these limits to

> adaptation will continue to play a negative role in attempts to address the problems seen today, perpetuating the negative trends tomorrow. (p. 410)

I used these reflections as I approached the government climate change strategies, curious about how limits and barriers to climate change adaptation may be framed through ableist ideologies. Wolbring (2009) notes that barriers and stressors unrelated to climate change can increase vulnerabilities to it, as they already reduce resiliency and adaptive capacities because of competing needs and limited resources. Indeed, the literature suggests that persons with disabilities are often physically, financially, and psychologically compromised, and yet, as I will demonstrate, they are still being asked to adapt and build resilience.

Vulnerability

Vulnerability is another contested term that pervades Canadian climate change strategies and responses. Vulnerability is defined in the glossary of terms by the IPCC (2012) as "the propensity or predisposition to be adversely affected" (p. 564) to climate change. The Fourth Assessment Report by the IPCC (2007) offered a little more insight into vulnerability as it defines it as follows:

> Vulnerability is the degree to which a system is susceptible to, and unable to cope with, adverse effects of climate change, including climate variability and extremes. Vulnerability is a function of the character, magnitude, and rate of climate change and variation to which a system is exposed, its sensitivity, and its adaptive capacity. (p. 883)

A working knowledge of these concepts is relevant to this study as the literature suggests that a principal goal of Canadian climate change adaptation strategies is to reduce vulnerabilities and build resilience (Alston & Whittenbury, 2010). Through immersing myself in the literature on vulnerable populations and climate change it became clear that everyone is being asked to adapt and build resilience, including communities who are already marginalized. While it is important to care for and protect everyone in the face of climatic threats, unbridled resilience thinking requires caution, as it often hides gross inequities. In fact, despite the recognition of the deeper vulnerabilities persons with disabilities have to climate change, policy makers pay little attention to disability within climate impact and adaptation strategies (Jodoin, Ananthamoorthy, & Lofts 2020).

As I journeyed through the climate change literature, I encountered several definitions and meanings that serve as useful background for conducting a thematic analysis. Ribot (2011) reminds us that words matter, that the term vulnerability requires that we ask why certain people are vulnerable and at risk and who is responsible for their vulnerabilities. When we simply ask people to adapt, we shift the focus from cause to response, rather than asking why people have to adapt in the first place (Ribot, 2011). Brooks, Adger, and Kelly (2005), state that "Vulnerability depends critically on context, and the factors that make a system vulnerable to a hazard will depend on the nature of the system and the type of hazard in question" (p. 152). In my preliminary review of the Canadian government climate change publications, it appeared as though the personal and contextual factors that make human systems vulnerable were not adequately considered. Early in my examination of these documents, I saw the Canadian government imposing substantial adaptation responsibilities on those whom they deemed to be vulnerable Canadians (such as persons with disabilities), without accounting for the broader systems that add to their burden of risks. Further, it seemed as though the government was only occasionally and generally speaking about vulnerability, without specifically including disability in these conversations. One example is that government climate change strategies ask vulnerable Canadians to increase resilience and adaptive capacities, while simultaneously reducing their individual carbon footprints. Ableism seems to be informing the strategies, for example, in carbon footprint discussions alone, as the Canadian government is calling for more people to walk, cycle, or take public transportation, without considering the accessibility and feasibility of each for persons with disabilities.

Brooks, Adger, and Kelly (2005) point out that even within the same country, vulnerability is socially and geographically differentiated and most often specific to local contexts (Brooks, Adger, & Kelly, 2005). They contend that it is 'people' not countries that are vulnerable and that local assessments must be carried out along with nation-wide research in order to appropriately understand vulnerability (Brooks, Adger, & Kelly, 2005). In my review of the literature, vulnerability emerged as a term that requires interrogation and explanation by both federal and local governments. By framing certain groups as vulnerable, policy makers could potentially compromise their agency while constructing and perpetuating hegemonic notions about these groups. While the scale of this MSW thesis does not allow me to put vulnerability at the forefront of my literature review and analysis, it remains a crucial term in climate strategy discussions, and as such, I speak to its importance at various points in my analytic journey.

Climate Resilience

Climate resilience is a term found in the Canadian Federal Government climate change publications, including within the letter I received from Canada's Minister of Environment and Climate Change. I introduce this term in my literature review for its widespread use in climate change strategies spanning human health and economy. Climate resilience is used both interchangeably and in tandem with adaptive capacity building in climate change adaptation strategies. The IPCC (2012) defines resilience as:

> The ability of a system and its component parts to anticipate, absorb, accommodate, or recover from the effects of a hazardous event in a timely and efficient manner, including through ensuring the preservation, restoration, or improvement of its essential basic structures and functions. (p. 563)

I note that this widely used definition does not speak specifically to human and social factors influencing resilience. Similarly, Nelson, Adger, and Brown (2007) have called for more scholarly discussions on the relationship between human resilience and adaptation within climate change research.

The concept of resilience has deep roots in the field of social work, with emerging critiques from this field as well as within human geography and political ecology. In their critique of resilience, MacKinnon and Derickson (2012) note that the term adaptation is derived from apolitical ecology and systems theories and has limited application to social structures. Similarly, in my review of adaptation literature, several emerging studies found that contextual politics and social systems often thwart or promote climate adaptation and climate resilience (Cameron, 2012; Noelke, et al., 2016; Mikulewicz, 2019). From the fields of climate resilient development and climate justice, Mikulewicz suggests that there are four key critiques of resilience thinking:

> Its inability to sufficiently recognize the large scale political, economic, and social forces affecting and effecting climate change. Its oversight of the analyzed systems' internal dynamics. The depoliticized, techno-managerial nature of resilience-

> centred solutions. The theoretical vagueness of resilience as applied by developmental actors. (p. 267)

I situate these critiques in my literature review as they help me to thoughtfully analyze the data I have chosen from interdisciplinary perspectives. Critical works such as this have helped to propel and float my own questions about climate strategies, adaptation, and persons with disabilities.

Swyngedouw and Heynen (2003) argue that akin to limits to adaptation across social dimensions, resilience thinking similarly privileges existing social structures and systems that are built upon injustice and uneven power relations. Further, Alam, et al. (2017) cite adaptation as being context-specific, with the ability for individuals and communities to adapt varying both within and across countries. Interestingly, when looking at biological limits to heat, sociologists have found that the effects of extreme heat are unevenly distributed across inequalities; for example, people with less education are least able to cope with the effects of extreme heat (Noelke et al., 2016). As I shared in my opening chapter, this research also connects to my own context and experience of disability, as I have been previously able to escape the extreme cold, heat, and humidity that flare my illnesses. At the same time, it is important for me to note that my experience of climate and illness is dynamic, as my physical health is better in British Columbia's temperate climate, yet most of my social support system resides in Nova Scotia. While Canadian government climate change literature speaks to an established need to adapt to a changing climate, few authors parse many of these concrete biological and social limits to adaptation. In a recent lecture on *climate change and social adaptation* at University of Victoria, Harvard Chair of Sociology Jason Beckfield (2020) explained that disasters create highly unequal experiences depending on the resources you have, spanning from financial to social networks. When considering the advantage private wealth has on mitigating the damaging effects of climate change, Beckwith (2020) notes that government health expenditures that prioritize public programs have the ability to even out this playing field. Similarly, Jones (2010) found that discrimination, social marginalization, and institutional inequities are well established as inhibitors of successful climate change adaptation. My review of the literature suggests that social barriers to adaptation often reflect the values and structures of a society, challenges that many scholars suggest will require systemic, political, and cultural shifts to solve (Hulme, et al., 2007).

Mikulewicz (2019) argues that resilience thinking fails to engage adequately with issues such as power and access to resources, or the possibility that increasing resiliency for some may conversely decrease it for others. In their analysis of resilience within social work literature, Park, Crath, and Jeffery (2018) found that the focus on building individual resilience is a process that often eclipses attention from the deep roots of structural oppressions. Similarly, resilience thinking cannot answer questions related to the inequality that we are seeing in climate adaptive processes, particularly in the Global South, where there are winners and losers in adaptive processes (Mikulewicz, 2019). Cameron (2012) contends that another critical oversight in adaptive processes to climate change is the exclusion of social, cultural, economic, political, and historical dynamics of colonization. It appears as though Canadian climate change strategies are positioned as politically neutral zones, where colonial power through ongoing practices such as resource extraction is rendered apolitical, as noted markedly by its absence from the strategies. As an example, Adger (2009) describes this playing out where limits to climate adaptation and resilience are analysed as a set of immutable thresholds in biology, economy, and technology. That is, limits to climate adaptation and resilience often fail to account for the ways in which our societies are constructed socially and politically (Adger, 2009). Similarly, Mikulewicz (2019) explains that adaptation in climate science is most often about building resilience rather than promoting social transformations through social justice, including decreasing existing vulnerabilities. In other words, resilience and adaptation are terms that appear to be "hijacked by the neoliberal development machine to consolidate capitalist expansion and cement the political and socio-economic status quo across multiple scales" (Mikulewicz & Taylor, 2019, p. 278). Calls for adaptation are situated within the urgency and panic surrounding climate change and my review of this particular corner of the literature suggests that climate concepts in the areas of adaptation, adaptive capacity, and climate resilience are inherently political and highly contested. I wrestle with some of these complexities in the chapters that follow.

Situating Social Work

Similar to the field of climate science itself, social work is a profession that calls us to wrestle with complexity, uncertainty, and risk. Erickson (2018) notes the ways in which social work is increasingly attentive to the injustices of environmental and climate change movements intertwined with the economic, social, and political realities of individuals. As such, social workers are now called to address both environmental and human inequities, since we are often unable to separate the two (Erickson, 2018). Similarly, Jef Peeters (2012) emphasizes "social work has a role to play in challenging the social, political, and economic structures and processes that cause climate change... this means that social work practices have to contribute to a great social transition, a systemic change" (p. 107). At the same time, Cumby (2016) reports that, although we are seeing an upswing in these conversations, social work has remained somewhat silent on issues such as climate change and the ways in which it is disproportionately affecting marginalized groups. In the literature that does exist, Cumby (2016) notes that due to their skills in capacity building, advocacy, and crisis response, social workers are already well-positioned to take on climate issues. Having said this, while social workers increasingly intervene in climate disasters by providing crisis responses (such as relocation, housing, food, and other social supports) they are less visible in climate change planning and policy (Alston, 2015). Furthermore, *The Routledge Handbook of Green Social Work* clearly illuminates the need for *green* social workers to play a role in shaping policy related to climate change, disasters, and other environmental issues (Dominelli, 2018).

While there is some literature that situates social work within climate change conversations, there is far less being said in the literature about the connections between disability, social work, and climate change. There are, however, some calls within other social science domains to bring a critical disability lens to climate change, underscoring the need to include disabled voices within climate change adaptation discourses, practices, and policies (Bell, Tabe, & Bell, 2020). When discussing the need for disability perspectives to be included within global climate change discussions, Bell, Tabe, and Bell suggest:

> A critical disability lens could foster climate change adaptation strategies that promote dignity and respect for embodied diversity, recognising people's capacities and skills rather than broadening existing health inequalities. (p. 685)

While the above research doesn't situate social work specifically, it does point to a more socially *just* approach to developing climate change strategies, one that includes disability perspectives. In the book *Climate Change Adaptation for Health and Social Services*, Walker and Mason (2015) note that there is limited research around the ways in which disabled people are impacted by climate change, with the exception of a small body of research from non-government organizations and United Nations agencies. In summary, the authors found that persons with disabilities lack a voice within climate change policymaking and that justice-oriented climate change initiatives must be tied to social issues and fields of social science (Walker & Mason, 2015). As a social worker, and a person with disabilities committed to climate justice, I felt called to address these inequities in my research.

CHAPTER THREE: Research Design

As a social worker committed to disability justice, social justice, and climate justice, I have chosen to examine six Canadian Federal Government climate change documents using a reflexive thematic analysis. In this chapter, I detail the theoretical framework and research design used to conduct a reflexive thematic analysis of these prominent climate change documents. In my journey to explore and extract themes from the data, I utilized justice-based guideposts from feminist disability studies and critical disability studies. In keeping with the reflexive nature of this study, I have utilized a social constructivist understanding of disability to establish this thesis. That is, my theoretical framework largely views disability as built around institutional and societal expectations of health and productivity. In addition, I bring a poststructural perspective to my framework and analysis, often borrowing from Foucault who was concerned with the production of meaning, power, and taken-for-granted knowledge. These perspectives largely inform my conceptual scaffold and analytical insights. In the sections that follow, I detail my reflexive thematic analysis research approach, expand upon my study's theoretical framework, present questions that guided my process, and introduce my six data sources.

Rationale for Reflexive Thematic Analysis

I chose to undertake a reflexive thematic analysis since this type of qualitative research allowed me to gather information in the form of *themes* from Canadian climate change documents. I draw upon this qualitative research approach for its resourceful, subjective, and reflexive nature, in which the researcher's subjectivity is viewed as a resource, rather than a hindrance to knowledge production (Gough & Madill, 2012; Braun & Clarke, 2019). Utilizing Braun and Clarke's reflexive approach to thematic analysis has given me the flexibility to narrate a story about the data through my own interpretive lens. Since reflexivity has been an integral part of my own research ethics, reflexive thematic analysis emerged as a natural fit for grounding my experiential knowledge throughout this process.

While later in this chapter I outline how I personalized reflexive thematic analysis, here I explain how I follow the broad and flexible guidelines offered by Victoria Clarke and Virginia Braun. In Braun and Clarke's (2006) early work, the authors described thematic analysis as follows:

> A method for identifying, analyzing and reporting patterns (themes) within data. It minimally organizes and describes your data in (rich) detail. However, frequently it goes further than this, and interprets various aspects of the research topic. (p. 79)

Known for its theoretical freedom, thematic analysis has often been described as foundational to qualitative research (Braun & Clarke, 2006; Nowell et al., 2017). Specifically related to my study, thematic analysis is also widely used in policy research (Herzog, Handke & Hitters, 2019).

More recently, three broad approaches predominate Braun et al.'s (2019) typology of thematic analysis: reflexive, reliability, and codebook. Reliability approaches tend to be more positivist, quantitative, and driven by demonstrations of coding reliability, while codebook approaches include more rigid definitions of themes and are based on a structured codebook (Braun, Clarke & Hayfield, 2019). Reflexive approaches, on the other hand, are influenced by a qualitative paradigm in which coding is seen as an evolving and organic process since the researcher engages with the data (Braun, Clarke, & Hayfield, 2019). As I began writing about and working with the data, it became clear that I could not remove my political positioning and interpretations from the analysis; thus, a reflexive research approach was a natural fit for the justice-focused research I wanted to undertake.

Reflexivity and Social Work Research

In the decade since Braun and Clarke (2006) first published their work, they have expanded their approach to thematic analysis to include the highly contextual *reflexivity* of the researcher (Braun & Clarke, 2019). As previously mentioned, this reflexive approach pairs well with qualitative studies in social work. Speaking on the merits of reflexivity in social work research, Probst (2015) states:

> Despite its "messiness" reflexivity remains a fundamental way, particularly in qualitative studies, to bolster credibility by parsing the research endeavor into its mutually affecting parts and documenting the pathways through which knowledge was generated. This is particularly critical in social work research, because decisions about policies and practices affecting the nation's most vulnerable populations rely heavily on the strength of research findings. Consumers of social work research, as well as those whom their work ultimately serves, should be able to trust the authenticity of the knowledge offered to them. The practice of reflexivity can support this aim. (p. 46)

In a similar way, reflexivity has allowed me to document the pathways through which knowledge was created in this study. As the above quote details, reflexive thematic analysis allows for a personal accountability that is crucial when researching with or about marginalized groups. Further, Jootun, McGhee, and Marland (2009) state that rigour cannot be measured by how well personal subjectivity has been controlled for, but it can be found where these personal and relational aspects of research are made apparent. Likewise, in their review of social work literature, Gringeri, Barusch, and Cambron (2013) cite reflexivity and theory as "twin pillars of rigorous qualitative research" (p. 61). By combining this documented importance of reflexivity in social work with the strengths of thematic analysis for analyzing policy documents, a reflexive qualitative approach is well suited to my research goals.

Inductive and Deductive Approaches to Thematic Analysis

Braun, Clarke, and Hayfield (2019) note that researchers doing a reflexive thematic analysis need to make a series of choices throughout their process, explaining why they have adopted each particular approach. Herzog, Handke, and Hitters (2019) explain that this transparency allows a researcher to not only increase their trustworthiness, but also clearly define the limitations of the knowledge they are producing. As such, the choice to pursue a more inductive versus deductive approach to my project is one of those key reflexive decisions.

Braun and Clarke (2018) explain that in an inductive framework you work from the bottom up, focusing on meaning while also remaining grounded in what comes out through the data; whereas a primarily deductive approach is a more theoretical orientation to the data in that preconceived questions drive your analysis. Having said this, they note that in reality, these two approaches are often muddled together, and our analyses are often a bit of both, tending primarily to one or the other in the design of a project (Braun & Clarke, 2018). While my approach to the data is primarily inductive, later in this chapter I outline some early queries that more deductively informed my analysis, questions that naturally emerged from my experiential and theoretical positioning. Inductively, I looked to the data unsure of what themes I might find, yet I was not without my own assumptions. For example, I went into this research knowing that persons with disabilities were not explicit collaborators in the development of federal climate change strategies in Canada. I assumed I would find these publications lacking in disability perspectives. While I was not sure of all that I would find in the data, my guiding questions do bring an element of deduction to the analytic process.

To the above point, I nonetheless utilized a primarily inductive approach when I explored the government climate change documents. While data-driven inductive approaches to reflexive thematic analysis are the most common, that is, driven by the data and *working up* from the data, they are not inductive in lacking a theoretical framework (Braun, Clarke, & Hayfield, 2019). In fact, reflexive thematic analysis invites and encourages theoretical consideration and sensitivity (Braun, Clarke, & Hayfield, 2019). For me, this means that my ontological and epistemological assumptions about disability and climate change cannot be removed from my research. Returning to the reflexive tenet of my research, I note that some theoretical assumptions introduced in my literature review are folded into the deductive queries that broadly inform this inductive research. As my reflexive thematic analysis is greatly influenced by my political and philosophical stance, in the sections that follow I outline these in greater detail.

Theoretical Framework

Feminist Disability Studies

My understandings of gender and disability have uniquely informed the ways in which I perceive the world. Specifically, through experiences of stigma and marginalization, I came to adopt a critical and feminist disability justice-focused politic. As articulated in my literature review, feminist disability studies unsettles stereotypes about disability by challenging our dominant assumptions about bodies and minds (Garland-Thomson, 2005). Further teasing out the usefulness of feminist disability studies, Garland-Thomson (2005) writes "like feminist studies itself, feminist disability studies is academic cultural work with a sharp political edge and a vigorous critical punch" (p.1557). At the same time, Grue (2011) suggests that, similar to social work and other fields with activist origins, feminist disability studies centres issues of social justice. The anti-oppressive focus in feminist disability studies therefore aligns with the justice-oriented goals of this research; thus, this political stance is built in to my research framework.

Since the fields of critical disability studies and feminist disability studies are often separated categorically and semantically, I highlight them separately for their individual contributions, while marrying them for their broader similarities. In illustrating their connections, Goodley (2016) argues that critical disability studies cannot analyze disability without recognizing the connections between the politics of gender, class, race, ethnicity, and sexuality. For these reasons, I have included critical, feminist, and intersectional theoretical orientations within my study's framework.

There is an emerging call for feminist disability theorists committed to social justice to step into the foreground of climate justice work. Indeed, many scholars underscore the need for feminist inquiries to confront climate change and the environmental crisis head-on (Macgregor, 2014; Oksala, 2018; Sachs, 2014). Oksala (2018) suggests that urgent issues such as climate change, energy justice, and food security require both feminist and ecological analyses, with feminist theorists called to form strong voices in developing environmental discussions. Yet, despite these calls to include feminist perspectives in the environmental movement, my literature review found that climate change research and strategies have largely excluded these voices. It is important to note that feminist disability studies does not simply add a disability perspective to a feminist analysis of climate change documents. According to Stienstra (2015):

> Feminist disability studies recognizes that by including and addressing the experiences of women and girls with disabilities, we transform feminist theory and practice to examine diverse embodiments as part of a range of humanity and illustrate experiences that are evident as well as those that are invisible and silenced. (p. 631)

As a female researcher and person with disabilities, this ethos is built into the format of both my reflexive analysis and the development of my literature review. Israel and Sachs (2012) have suggested that feminist scholars engaged in climate research should take seriously claims from climate science, while also examining the social and political aspects of that knowledge and practice. I join this growing body of research not to dispute climate change phenomena but to shine a light on social implications that spring from these politicized climate change and adaptation strategies. In *Only Resist: Feminist Ecological Citizenship and the Post-politics of Climate Change*, Sherilyn Macgregor (2014) states:

> Even if we can question the grand claim of a universal climate consensus, I would argue that the value of the post-political theoretical framework lies in its tools for problematizing the widely accepted environmentalist discourses (for example, of "behavior change" and "resilience") that sustain elite neoliberal interests. (p. 629)

This quote helps to situate the importance of critical, politicized analyses within environmental science, including climate change. Further, other feminist authors have highlighted the need to problematize resilience and other taken-for-granted terms in climate change strategies. Hall (2017) notes that environmental and climate justice literature informs us that addressing these issues is not only about consulting scientific and economic experts, but also about attending to injustices that operate in the background, often out of sight.

A reflexive thematic analysis allows me to stay grounded in a critical feminist disability politic, while still being receptive to what I might find in the climate change strategies. Feminist scholars have highlighted the utility of feminist approaches for challenging calls to individual responsibility, as well as calling for more intersectional approaches to global issues. Carolyn Sachs (2014) contends that there is a pressing need for more disability scholars, feminists, and activists to take up climate change as a central issue in their fields of work. I have attempted to answer this call in the work of my thesis.

Feminist disability studies aligns with my research goals because of its movement toward activism and social change. Rosemarie Garland-Thomson (2001) reminds us that feminist disability studies is often concerned with interpreting bodily variations, the relationship between bodies and their environments, and the practices that produce both the disabled and temporarily able-bodied. Garland-Thomson (2001) further explains that the attention to activism in feminist disability studies shifts the focus away from the pathologizing of women's bodies, the body's abilities, and the politics of appearance. Similarly, Johnson (2017) notes the ways in which feminism highlights how sexism shows up in disability, differentially impacting women and men. Indeed, a feminist approach to research regards truth as contextualized within lived experiences of gendered oppression (Moosa-Mitha, 2015). Consequently, I take my lead from Johnson (2017), who suggests that bridging feminist disability studies with environmental justice and intersectionality calls us to consider the power dynamics that privilege bodies who fit within a narrow view of normal, a view that both constricts and confines us. Indeed, feminist voices need to move out from the margins and intersectional issues (such as race, class, and gender) need to be a central focus within climate change issues (Sachs, 2014).

Critical Disability Studies

I wish to make clear that my theoretical framework is grounded in critical understandings of disability and ableism. These understandings of bodies and minds are sometimes, but not always, located within feminist-disability studies. Since this is a reflexive analysis, I want to shed light on a few of my assumptions. For example, Goodley (2016) greatly informs my understandings of critical disability studies in the following:

> Critical disability studies start with disability but never end with it: disability is *the* space from which to think though a host of political, theoretical, and practical issues that are relevant to all. (p. 157)

In this way, critical disability studies offers up a perspective that acknowledges the vast contextual experiences of those located at the margins, which are not limited to intersections of sex and gender. From this viewpoint, disability is mutable and highly personal, yet there are also many ways in which those who are seen as disabled are disadvantaged, stigmatized, and othered. From this place, ableism emerges as a broad term to describe active social and institutional oppressions that control and subjugate persons with disabilities. Indeed, ableism speaks to varied, heterogeneous experiences stemming from ableist normativity.

My politics also align with those of Withers (2012), who views disability and ableism as a socially constructed phenomenon that intersects with other systems of oppression, such as colonialism and racism. From a critical disability perspective, ableism is an important concept to consider when producing strategies that impact human health and well-being, since it shapes the ways in which we view the value of life, productivity, and health (Storey, 2007). Similarly, bodies and the body politic are interlocked and "we must consider the ways that ableism functions at the discursive, rhetorical and material levels" (Dingo, 2007, p. 105). Critical disability studies that center ableism have also emerged from findings across many disciplines (Campbell, 2009; Wolbring, 2009, 2012). That is, ableism appears in law, medicine, sociology, and religion, with healthy citizens regarded as normative, autonomous, reasonable, and rational beings for which societies are built (Goodley & Lawthorn, 2019). As Goodley and Lawthorn (2019) state, "as good poststructuralists, we already knew that disability relied on its opposite – ability – in order to exist" (p. 234). Goodley (2016) further illustrates the field's usefulness for my poststructural analysis of climate change data when he notes that critical disability studies is mindful of late capitalism, neoliberalism, as well as the impacts of local, national, and international economic realities on the lives of persons with disabilities. Critical disability studies is likewise attentive to intersectionality and the complexities inherent in contemporary times, which attunes it nicely to the uneven consequences of climate change.

Reflexively, I underpin these theoretical and political elements within this study since they are integral to my personal and professional beliefs and practices. As a social worker and person with disabilities, I constantly aim to resist and challenge ableism and injustices that stem from beliefs about non-normative bodies and minds. While I view the climate change strategies through an inductive data-driven analysis, I am curious about how they frame health and disability since I cannot separate my feminist and critical disability politics from my analysis.

An Intersectional Approach

Gaard (2015) suggests that intersectional, feminist voices and experiences should be at forefront of urgent global issues. Further underscoring this call, feminist scholars Israel and Sachs (2012) note that intersections of race, ethnicity, gender, and economic status position people and their environment differentially. I include an intersectional approach within my theoretical framework as it aligns with critical disability studies in ways that I have already highlighted. As Goodley (2016) suggests, critical disability studies may begin with centering disability but these issues "inevitably become interconnected with the politics of class, gender, sex/uality, race, and ethnicity" (p. 233).

Relatedly, in the article *Climate Change through the lens of intersectionality*, Kaijser and Kronsell (2013) offer the following questions for researchers engaged in intersectional theoretical approaches to climate change to reflect upon:

> Which social categories, if any, are represented in the empirical material? Which social categories are absent? Are there any observable explicit or implicit assumptions about social categories and about relations between social categories? What identities are promoted and considered to serve as grounds for political action? Are any other aspects of identity neglected or deemed insignificant? (p. 430)

I connect these questions to the politics of my study, as the authors note that intersectionality is grounded in feminist understandings of knowledge and power and that analytically these perspectives can help to shed light on how systems of power interact and interrelate (Kaijser & Kronsell, 2013). I use the above queries to better understand and situate intersectionality within my feminist, critical disability justice-oriented research. Taking the lead from anti-oppressive feminist scholars, I look to intersectional approaches to help me situate and discuss the power structures at play within climate change strategies. I move forward with the understanding that studies that focus on only one variable or challenge, fail to consider how inequality is reinforced intertwined with multiple structures of domination (Kaijser & Kronsell, 2013).

Sachs (2014) notes that an intersectional approach is used to unmask inequalities in research done by critical race scholars, feminist scholars, and more recently by scholars in geography and agriculture. These researchers highlight the significance of overlapping systems of oppression in the face of food insecurity and environmental disasters (Sachs, 2014). At the same time, Steinstra (2015) explains that many disability studies have been criticized for lacking reflexivity, particularly around issues related to race, ethnicity, and whiteness. Stienstra (2015) suggests that to "analyze and engage using intersectionality requires thinking about inclusion and exclusion, distribution of resources, manifestations of global inequalities such as racism, ableism, colonialism, and sexism, as well as systems and structures used to maintain inequalities" (p. 632). Many persons with disabilities are also located at the intersection of other oppressions, compounding their experiences of environmental racism and/or other social injustice. In my literature review, I found that these varied, intersectional perspectives are not at the fore of climate change discussions.

McCruer (2006) notes that a disability justice-oriented approach to research pairs well with intersectional and feminist perspectives as it recognizes the importance of disability within other identities and sites of historical marginalization. For example, Mia Mingus (2011) writes about her experiences as a queer, disabled, woman of colour, who does not often see environmental or disability activists who reflect her positioning, and rarely observes spaces that address disability while connecting it with other issues. Mingus (2011) imagines activism spaces that are less segregated, more accessible, places that do not further isolate disabled communities. That said, at the outset of my thesis journey I attended community groups held by *Joyful Resistance*, workshops in the areas of decolonizing environmental activism and anti-oppressive practice facilitated by BIPOC (Black, Indigenous, People of Colour) activists. These learning circles helped me to reflect on the diverse voices that are missing from Canadian climate change strategies, as well as those who are absent from my own research project.

Situating Foucault

Adding to the feminist and critical disability focused theoretical blueprint I highlighted above, Diamond and Quinby (1988) note the usefulness of using Foucauldian thought as a way to deconstruct what is portrayed as normal and natural while also exposing the workings of the power-knowledge nexus. This theme of deconstructing what is thought to be natural has particular relevance to my study, as normal is routinely equated to natural, good, and better. This normalcy is a conceptual tool, often deployed as hegemonic ideals of bodies and minds, a compulsory able-bodiedness so to speak (St. Pierre, 2017). While many climate change documents do not explicitly mention disabled people, Lennard Davis (2013) explains that even in texts that do not center disability, issues of normalcy are fully deployed. Similarly, in their book, *Gramsci, Space, Nature, Politics*, Ekers, et al. (2012) highlight the work of Antonio Gramsci and his notions of hegemony - that is, leadership and dominance of certain groups over others. Ekers et al. (2012) expand on Gramsci's ideas of class, social difference, and racialization within geopolitical movements by bridging some of the theoretical work of Gramsci and Foucault. Bridging together biopolitics and hegemony, St. Pierre (2017) refers to hegemony as:

> The impulse toward a seamless order without interruption. It is only by regulating the desires and relations of the working class within every sphere of life that capitalism can generate consent and reproduce itself – as if it were the only option. The last part is essential to the operation of hegemony, since like compulsory able-bodiedness, capitalism offers a choice when there actually is none. (p. 345)

Similarly, in drawing connections to bio-politics and capitalism in this study, I used reflexive thematic analysis as a means by which to search for the hegemony in the climate change strategies, pointing to the diffuse and active exercises of power. I look to the data see how dominant, influential norms are impressed upon bodies and minds.

Governmentality and Responsibilization. Michel Foucault coined the term *governmentality* and its related analysis to describe a way of governing that focuses on mechanisms of rule with regard to problems and solutions and the "techniques that are employed to put these solutions into effect" (Wakefield & Fleming, 2009, p. 2). Linking these practices to climate change, Watts (2011) characterizes adaptation and resilience building as green governmentality, where a new ecology of rule is perpetuated through capitalism and neoliberalism, what he calls "maladaptation" (p. 88). These processes are relevant to my study as I am concerned with the productive and cyclical nature of ableism in climate change strategies, including the ways in which persons with disabilities are governed and the ways in which they are governing themselves. For these reasons, I reference governmentality for its usefulness in analyzing "demonstrable plans and formal procedures" within official documents (Wakefield & Fleming, 2009, p. 3).

Closely aligned with the process of governmentality is the related act of responsibilization. Wakefield and Fleming (2009) describe responsibilization as a neoliberal strategy that was conceptualized in the governmentality literature of the mid-1990's. Responsibilization is an important component of my theoretical framework, as it refers to the ways in which accountability is turned back to individuals and communities to govern their own risks (Schirato, Danaher, & Webb, 2012). Some feminist scholars have already touched on how neoliberal processes of responsibilization are showing up in climate change documents, as we are being asked to change our behaviours without questioning the institutional inequalities and capitalist regimes that have led to environmental crisis (Macgregor, 2014; Rose, 1999). While I was developing this study, I could not help but wonder how responsibilization might be playing out where persons with disabilities are rendered reliant on government assistance and healthcare, yet, when confronting the climate, they are asked to adapt and self-manage the risks.

The *Doing* of Reflexive Thematic Analysis

Now that I have outlined my theoretical framework, I will move on to the *doing* of reflexive thematic analysis with an inductive approach. Braun and Clarke (2019) note that this type of qualitative research is organic, iterative, flexible, and exploratory, allowing for more personal interpretations of their prescribed methods. As Willig (2008) reflects, thematic analysis is less like a recipe and more like an adventure. That being said, in 2006, Braun and Clarke published a widely used guide to thematic analysis that outlined a six-step approach to data analysis. While I have moved through the data using these as a guideline, I am also reflexive and transparent about when and where my own theoretical and creative approaches were utilized.

Braun and Clarke's (2006) six steps to thematic analysis include: becoming familiar with the data; generating codes; searching for themes; reviewing these themes; defining the themes; and writing-up an analysis of the data. Yet, as I have highlighted, since that time the authors have expanded and developed their approach to thematic analysis to include the context specific *reflexivity* of the researcher and their process (Braun & Clarke, 2009). Researcher 'positioning' and underlying assumptions are always a part of qualitative research and reflexivity is crucial to unpacking and understanding these (Braun & Clarke, 2019). As such, I have been reflexive with the ways in which my process and analysis has been drawn from my personal experience and theoretical positioning.

Familiarisation

The widely accepted starting point for reflexive and other types of thematic analysis is familiarisation, meaning a thorough and repeated reading of the data for an intensive immersion with the content (Braun, Clarke, & Hayfield, 2019). According to Braun and Clarke (2006) "immersion usually involves repeated reading of the data and reading the data in an active way – searching for meanings and patterns" (p. 87). Thus, I read and reread the six documents several times each, flagging where health, illness, vulnerability, and disability were both included and excluded. I made detailed notes and highlights around recurring passages and began to move these into separate documents. Logging these discursive findings in a series of journals was accessible and adaptive in itself, since recovering from a concussion my computer usage and visual capacities were limited. This manageable research approach allowed me to index locations in the data where persons with disabilities were referenced, so I could return to these places and begin to make sense of the underlying themes and meanings. Not only was this approach accessible and organic for me, memo writing has been of use for many qualitative researchers employing thematic analysis (Herzog, Handke, & Hitters, 2019). Herzog, Handke, and Hitters (2019) also contend that memo-writing and note-taking is linked to quality control, as it supports an active engagement with the data and often helps to promote self-reflexivity.

To aid in my process of becoming familiar with the data, I pinned the *Adapting to a Changing Climate* (Government of Canada, 2016a) poster on the wall above my computer desk. Over a period of fourteen months, I kept returning to the text and images, each time reflecting from a greater depth of critical inquiry and experiential knowledge. While I read the documents, I made journal notes about each and copied pieces of the texts verbatim. This immersion in the data allowed me to make note of patterns that eventually became latent and semantic codes. I engaged in regular, thorough, and illustrative discussions with my thesis committee on several codes and early themes that emerged. Based on suggestions offered by my occupational therapist and physician, I avoided computer screens in my initial concussion recovery, and purposefully reread the printed chapters of my data sources while making handwritten notes on each. At times, I used a text-to-speech feature that would read the data aloud to me. To help me begin to generate codes, in a separate journal I logged the location and number of times where the terms adaptation, adaptive capacity, resilience, health, disability, and vulnerability were used and what was being said at each instance.

Figure 1

Journal Excerpt

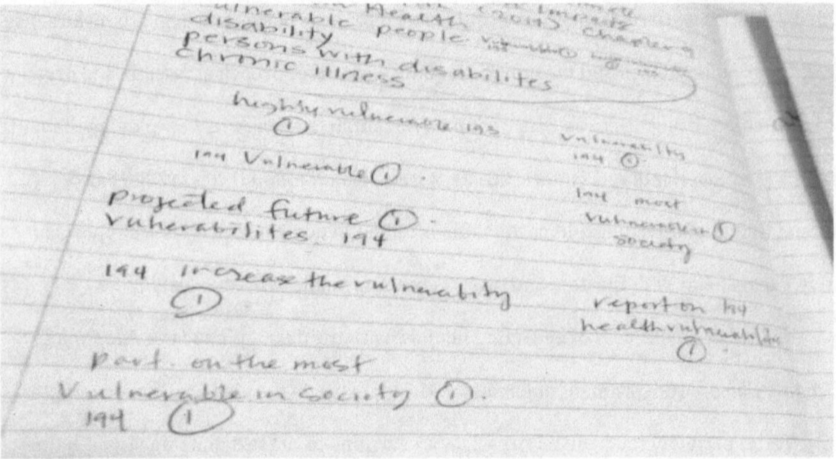

[IMAGE DESCRIPTION: An image of ruled white paper featuring blue ink handwriting, with reoccurring terms and page numbers extracted from the data sources, including instances of the terms vulnerability, highly vulnerable, most vulnerable in society, and increases in vulnerability.]

Note. A photograph of a page in the journal I used for tracking the key terms within my thematic analysis.

This photo offers a glimpse into my thematic analysis process and the personalized system I used for tracking the location and underlying meanings of recurring terms. I read through my data sources making codes around where, how, and why terms like health, disability, adaptation, adaptive capacity, resilience, chronic illness, and vulnerability appeared while examining the underlying meanings behind each occurrence. This personal and reflexive analytical strategy was adaptive in itself, as when I was recovering from a concussion and unable to spend long periods of time on a computer screen, I could contemplate codes and connections and deduce meaning from the items I had extracted on these hand-written entries.

Coding

Braun, Clarke, and Hayfield (2019) note that coding is always a subjective process and I have found this to be true. Although I looked to the data inductively to discover what themes were waiting to be extracted, I proceeded with some general questions in mind. In a following section, I highlight with greater reflexivity the questions I considered and the theoretical framework from which they sprang. In saying this, the one overarching question was: how is health and disability showing up in Canadian climate change strategies? This helped narrow my search for codes as I was drawn to sections of the data that contained reference to health, illness, vulnerability, and disability (to name a few).

When I began coding, I found what I believed to be themes emerging from the data, only to later understand that themes are generally broader than codes, and that several codes would eventually lead me to a single theme. For example, I would often see in the data that climate change was being framed as *causing* illness and disability and while these assumptions were frequently coded, they eventually pointed me to a larger, central theme, i.e., the overall exclusion and omission of persons with disabilities and pre-existing illness from climate change strategies. Although in a deductive sense, I had a hunch this would be the case, by becoming intimately acquainted with the data through coding, themes started to appear in a more inductive way. I developed several codes from reviewing my six data sources, as there were many recurring statements and viewpoints. I labelled each while collating them on electronic and paper files. Flagging these repetitions as codes and mapping them across all six data sources allowed me to assess the material in a cohesive, meaningful way, eventually leading to themes. This is where conversations with my supervisory team became very useful, by thoughtfully working through the codes and further demarcating the themes that I discovered.

Engaging with my theoretical framework, I approached the data set as Graham (2011) suggests, looking to statements "not so much for what they say but what they *do*; that is, one questions what the constitutive or political effects of saying this instead of that might be" (p. 667). Moving forward, "the objective is to explicate statements that function to place a discursive frame around a particular position; that is, statements which coagulate and form rhetorical constructions that present a particular reading of social texts" (Graham, 2011, p. 667). In the same way, my research procedures included reading the texts for statements about health, bodies, and minds. I would flag certain statements and sections that spoke about bodies and health conditions, and how each are situated within the climate change strategies. In a series of journals, I collated statements that helped elucidate how and why certain aspects of health are included and the functions that these statements serve. Through this process of reading, re-reading, and journaling, it became apparent that certain statements were repeated often throughout all of the data sources and these became very clear, clustered codes.

Themes and Review

After generating codes, the development and reviewing of themes was a considerable task. This phase involved a thoughtful process of sorting codes from themes, often cited as a tricky endeavour in thematic analysis as researchers often mistake codes for themes (Braun & Clarke, 2006). Initially, I had come up with about seven separate themes, including a number of clear inconsistencies and contradictions in the data. As an example, I felt as though contradictions were a strong enough theme on their own, however, after spending time reviewing themes with my supervisory committee this finding remained a code that was best described in the context of broader data meanings.

As Braun, Clarke, and Hayfield (2019) suggest, I spent a considerable amount of time refining my themes, cycling through several iterations and interpretations of each. In Clarke's (2017) YouTube lecture *What is thematic analysis*, themes are described as similar to storybooks, an interpretive, creative telling of a story through the researcher's personal lens. As Braun and Clarke (2006) suggest, it was useful for me to conceptualize themes as small stories that connect to a larger story.

After refining the themes that captured my conceptualization of the data set, I returned to the data and compared my themes against particular sections of the six documents. The purpose of this was to gain clarity and credibility for each theme. Some themes were discarded, while more often they were combined to create a larger more illustrative theme. This process is often labelled as *refining the themes* and for me it meant checking back with my data set to be sure they were in fact telling the 'story' that I had inferred.

Defining and Naming Themes

Defining and naming themes was the next logical move, and it also happens to be the next phase in Braun and Clarke's (2006) six-step process. This step involved formulating a descriptive *storybook* highlight of the most important themes and how they help make sense of the data. Braun and Clarke (2019) note that their orientation to themes is not typically a taken-for-granted, obvious or blatant summary of the data. In reflexive thematic analysis, themes come out of patterns of shared meanings, often united by a core concept, or central organizing concept (Braun & Clarke, 2019). This emphasis on patterns of shared meaning marries well with my critical and poststructural approach to the data, as my themes were more latent findings rather than an overtly semantic or surface summary. My theoretical orientation and extensive literature review allowed me to mull over the data in an informed, intensive, and judicious capacity.

The process of meaning making was long and winding and did not always proceed in a linear fashion (as is often the case with theme development). Initially, I had kept the main themes very succinct, yet, after reading and listening to how others have used thematic analysis, it was clear that a rich, descriptive theme would best help to summarize my findings. My themes were defined, constructed, named, and re-named over a period of several months with the data. These theme iterations were also born out of thoughtful discussions with my supervisory committee, as they were not only worked through on computer and paper, they were shared and reflected back dialogically through committee interaction. In my analysis, I also link back to some of the terms and definitions from my literature review as they helped to contextualize my findings. For this process, I have partly relied on the poststructural research scaffold set forth by Graham (2011) who states, "language is the tool through which people communicate ideas, and successful communication between individuals and especially groups of individuals relies on the definition and specification that language allows" (p. 668). My themes were defined and refined through my theoretical framework, methods, and supervisory conversations.

Producing the Research

The final step in a thematic analysis is the *proof in the pudding* so to speak. This phase involves writing up my analysis of the data, and more broadly, the thesis in its entirety. Reflexively, this step was similar to the other five in that it was interactive and cyclical, rather than linear. As Nowell et al. (2017) remark, thematic analysis is iterative and reflective, often requiring back and forth movements between steps. As an example, I began writing at a very early stage to aid in my familiarisation and synthesis of the data. During meetings with my supervisory committee, we interrogated the more latent findings in the data, and I presented patterns as they materialized. Early on, I began to identify several cyclic themes in the strategies, including where, how, and why certain recurring terms were used in each particular strategy. Rather than include each as a theme, they began to take shape as sub-themes under broader more exhaustive headings. Indeed, this process of working and re-working with the data included steep learning curves and thoughtful engagement with my methodology and data. In the end, I return to guidance from Braun and Clarke (2019) who state that quality thematic analysis is not a practice that involves following procedures correctly, rather, it is more about the researchers own thoughtful and reflective engagement with the data.

Guiding Questions

Although my approach to thematic analysis was primarily inductive (in that I went into the data unsure about what I might find) my analytical journey was also guided by some early foundational questions. This is not unlike other studies that use thematic analysis, where there is often a deductive component to an inductive research process (Braun & Clarke, 2017; Braun & Clarke, 2019). Part of the reflexive component of my thematic analysis is that I began the study with a hunch about what I might find in the data, given my experiential knowledge and early readings. This reflexivity extends to how I even came to question climate change and persons with disabilities, as I am situated both as a researcher and as a person whose health is greatly impacted by government policies and strategies.

Along with being curious about what I would uncover using a primarily inductive approach, and in keeping with my commitment to feminist, critical, and intersectional methodological approaches, I did reflect on some general guiding questions. As I highlighted in my literature review, my theoretical framework is influenced by the work of Alison Kafer. Kafer's expertise includes the areas of feminist and queer theory, race and ethnicity studies, disability studies, and environmental justice. To help expose systemic oppressions and structural inequalities in marginalized communities, Kafer (2013) calls us to ask the following three questions: "how has disability been depoliticized, removed from the realm of the political, which assumptions and definitions of disability facilitate this removal, and what are the effects of such de-politicization" (p. 10)? I have used these questions both as jumping off points as well as anchors, as they help to situate my analysis in broader calls for social justice. I come back to these queries throughout my data analysis and again in my discussion chapter.

As mentioned, Braun and Clarke (2018) have provided a six-step process to thematic analysis while at the same time encouraging a creative, contextualized, and flexible approach in terms of both methods and theoretical underpinnings. Although I have been guided by their six-step process, this study is influenced by their later work around reflexive thematic analysis which asks the researcher to let go of any prescriptive rules. By developing a list of personal reflective questions, I am able to bring forth my theoretical positioning while at the same time giving myself tangible guideposts to return to and consider. While I read the data looking for themes inductively, the questions below have also helped to guide me through this thesis, creating a path toward understanding where, how, and why health and disability appear in the data.

1) How do health and disability appear in the documents? Where? Why?
2) Who is benefiting from Canadian climate change strategies?
3) How is justice for persons with disabilities governed by the strategies?
4) How is justice for persons with disabilities constrained by the strategies?
5) Is the Canadian government preparing health professionals (social workers) for the unique needs of persons with disabilities and chronic illness in the face of climate change?

These are the principal questions that brought me to this area of research. Starting with and returning to these foundational queries helped me to navigate and ground this study in an overarching commitment to disability justice. These questions further facilitated a *stirring of the ground* so to speak, as I will outline later, they prompted me to challenge taken-for-granted assumptions about bodies, minds, health, and disability in the data.

Data Selection

I carefully chose these key publications based on a number of factors outlined below. Firstly, official documents and policies offer critical insights into social practices and institutional structures (Gilson, et al., 2018; Jóhannesson, 2010). As such, the documents I have chosen allowed me to explore how health and disability are portrayed in Canadian Federal Government climate change strategies. Furthermore, I selected these six Canadian climate change documents for my study based on the following reflexive criteria:

- My personal concerns/research questions that led me to this thesis topic
- The saliency of the documents, primarily as defined by Canada's Minister of Environment and Climate Change the Honourable Catherine McKenna
- The scope of my MSW thesis and the time that I had for data analysis

Because I was particularly curious about the ways in which ableism might be dominating this new terrain of climate change strategies, I searched for documents that were highlighted as accessible, and that could be found online through Canadian government websites. My aim was also to analyze documents that the Federal Government of Canada positions as the most relevant and timely regarding persons with disabilities and climate change. This mode of inquiry was both personal and political, as like myself, many persons with chronic illness attain information via the internet and social media. In this way, I was not only a researcher in this study, I was also a citizen with chronic illness acquiring information about how climate change could impact my well-being and what measures might mitigate potential harm. Through my own web search, I found several documents that would be accessed for health-related climate change information by federal/provincial climate change planners as well as Canadians at large. Fittingly, my research questions led me to discover the same collection of government climate change publications that were later recommended to me through official government correspondence.

In addition to a preliminary literature review, I emailed Canada's Minister of Environment and Climate Change the Honourable Catherine McKenna to ask what government documents would be appropriate given the scope of my interests. Catherine McKenna is a Canadian Liberal Party politician who was appointed to the new role of Canadian Minister of Environment and Climate Change by Prime Minister Justin Trudeau in 2015. I contacted the Minister twice via email and did not receive a reply over a period of approximately five months. I am fortunate to have a friend who works for the Liberal Party of Canada, and he suggested that I reach out via social media (Facebook and Twitter). After sending two messages this way I received a prompt reply to my earlier email. I have included this response letter from the Minister in Appendix A. It is important to note, in my emails and messages to the Honourable Catherine McKenna I did not ask for *adaptation* specific climate change strategies. Specifically, I asked what Canadian climate change strategies, supports, and publications would be most applicable to persons with disabilities and vulnerable populations. As you can see in her response letter, from the first sentence and throughout most paragraphs, adaptation was presented to me as most relevant to climate change and persons with disabilities. Indeed, adaptation and climate resilience are presented as not only one of the four pillars of the Pan-Canadian Framework on Clean Growth and Climate Change, but also as foundational to many of other climate change strategies and documents. Curiously, in my messages to the Minister I mentioned that I am a person with disabilities and that my study was related to persons with disabilities three times, and only once did I reference vulnerable Canadians. Concerning this, I call attention to the two-page response where persons with disabilities are only explicitly mentioned once and she sweepingly references and conflates them with vulnerable populations. Carrying forward my literature review reference to Alice in Wonderland and proverbial rabbit holes, the Minister's response and the slight manipulation of my question only made me curiouser and curiouser. Of course, this could be a generic, form letter that is frequently sent to people with similar questions, either way, this official government letter provided confirmation I was using the most relevant data for my analysis.

Data Sources

To validate my data selection, I note that the climate documents I had previously discovered on my own were included in the letter I received from Canada's Minister of

Environment and Climate Change. From her suggestions, I selected a total of six documents as data sources for this project. I chose these items for the following reasons:

a) They each speak to the health of Canadians from a broad scope.

b) They included several documents I found in my preliminary research around climate strategies for persons with disabilities in Canada.

c) Their inclusion as suggested readings from Canada's Minister of Environment and Climate Change flagged them as relevant timely documents related to the questions I wanted answered.

Two of the six documents are chapters found in a 286-page report titled *Canada in a Changing Climate: Sector Perspectives on Impacts and Adaptation* (Warren & Lemmen, 2014), and represent scientific assessments published by Natural Resources Canada. On the second page of her letter, the Minister made note that *Human Health* (Chapter 7) and *Adaptation: Linking Research and Practice* (Chapter 9) may be of particular interest. I initially chose to include Chapter *7: Human Health* by Berry, et al. (2014) as it was one of a few recent public government publications that specifically addressed human health and vulnerable populations. Later it was also suggested to me by Canada's Minister of Environment and Climate Change, confirming its usefulness for this study. This publication is available in English on the Government of Canada's Natural Resources website. The 41-page, full colour, PDF chapter is introduced as being led by Natural Resources Canada, with the involvement of over 90 authors and 115 expert reviewers and is said to have been a synthesis of over 1500 recent publications (Government of Canada, 2019). The authors are employees of Health Canada and the Public Health Agency of Canada and the chapter includes contributions from authors associated with Environment Canada, Health Canada,

Public Health Agency of Canada, Centre for Coastal Health and one Environmental Consultant (energy policy researcher). The chapter is divided into 7 sections including key findings and references, including several tables, figures, boxes and case studies with English text. This document does not contain descriptive images and English appears to be the only available language format.

Chapter 9 is extracted from the same larger document as the previous chapter, *Canada in a Changing Climate: Sector Perspectives on Impacts and Adaptation* (Warren & Lemmen, 2014). This 33-page chapter is titled *Adaptation, Linking Research and Practice*, and focuses primarily on adaptation with an emphasis on synthesizing research and recommending a number of adaptation activities (Eyzaguirre & Warren, 2014). With complementary examples related to my areas of interest, the authors include reference to an understanding of barriers and challenges to adaptation, noting the need to augment adaptive capacities in order for adaptation measures to succeed (Eyzaguirre & Warren, 2014). This chapter highlights that much of the adaptation action at present is focused on capacity building, planning, policy and raising awareness. Several human factors are also considered, factors said to help expedite the pace between adaptation awareness and action, such as, effective champions, strong leaders, supportive strategies and policies (Eyzaguirre & Warren, 2014). This chapters focus on adaptation in climate research and practice (along with its recommendation by Canada's Minister of Environment and Climate Change) makes it an ideal data source for my project.

Related to these two chapters, I have included the poster *Adapting to Our Changing Climate in Canada* (Government of Canada, 2016a), as an additional mixed media data source. The poster was designed using information from the report, *Canada in a Changing*

Climate: Sector Perspectives on Impacts and Adaption (Warren & Lemmen, 2014) which is the sizeable document from which the two previously highlighted chapters are drawn. The paragraph that precedes the poster states that they (the government) have worked with subject matter experts in governments, universities and non-government organizations to produce what they call current, relevant and accessible sources of information. This poster synthesizes and simplifies information found in the cited scientific assessments with the intended audience cited as being the general public, educators and community groups. The poster features simple visuals and short summaries of government data on climate change and adaptation. This document was the most accessible to me from home as I began my research as it was markedly highlighted in English text on the Government of Canada website. In fact, this poster was the first government climate change publication that I found, and it centers adaptation as a critical response to climate threats. Initially I could not read the small and blurry English text as it appeared on the website, but I was able to order two free copies in the mail through an online form. Along with Figure 2 below, I have added an image description, an important accessibility tool for persons who are visually impaired.

Figure 2

Poster: Adapting to our Changing Climate in Canada

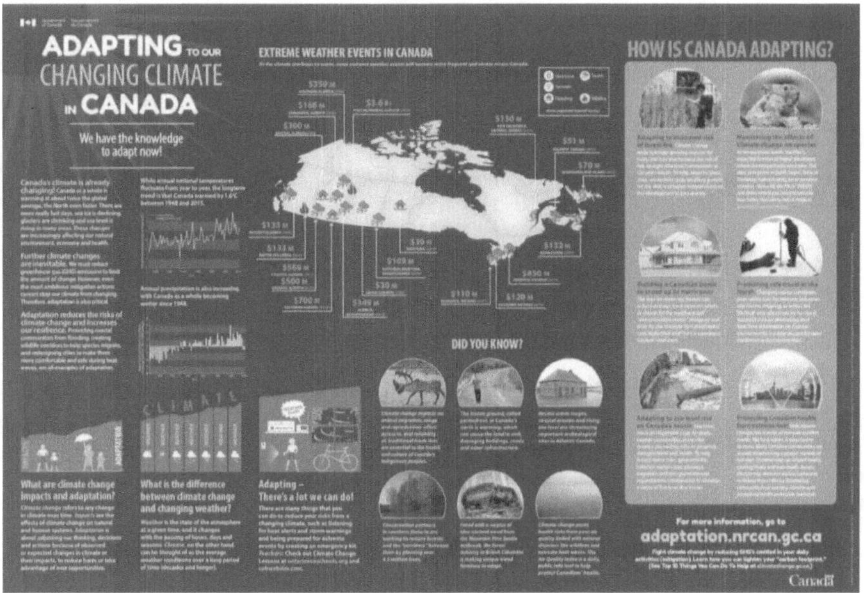

[IMAGE DESCRIPTION: A green infographic poster titled "Adapting to our Changing Climate in Canada," produced by the government of Canada. the infographic includes a yellow map of Canada as the centre figure, pink text boxes below with cartoon images of a person standing with a flashlight, a bicycle and four more white and yellow coloured cartoon people standing, one holding an umbrella. The right side of the poster includes twelve small photographs, three photos include images of people, two men are standing in their distinct image and in another one is standing while one is laying on the ice measuring its thickness. additional photos of animals, trees, water, houses, cities, and infrastructure correspond to short captions about climate change and adaptation in Canada.]

Note. The above figure is a poster retrieved from Government of Canada Climate Change Publications (2016a) website.

As you can see in her letter, McKenna pointed me to published reports by Health Canada and the Public Health Agency of Canada that include "guidelines and frameworks to assess and reduce climate risks in vulnerable populations" (p.2). That being the case, I included two of the most relevant documents in this list as further data sources: *Climate Change Impacts on the Health of Canadians* (2017) and *Human Health in a Changing Climate: A Canadian Assessment of Vulnerabilities and Adaptive Capacity* (2008). These documents were new to me and not ones that I found in my preliminary web search for relevant Canadian climate change publications.

Climate Change Impacts on the Health of Canadians (2017) is a 30-page document highlighted as a science narrative from the Public Health Agency of Canada. It is offered online in English as a PDF and in the fine print it says that upon request it can be made available in alternate formats. Throughout the five text-based chapters, health impacts of climate change are explored across dimensions that include chronic disease, mental health, infectious disease, food safety, water borne disease, extreme weather and physical activity. The second chapter is my primary focus as it specifically addresses adaptation measures and strategies to protect health with climate impacts and vulnerabilities being considered.

My fifth data source is *Human Health in a Changing Climate: A Canadian Assessment of Vulnerabilities and Adaptive Capacity* (Public Health Agency of Canada, 2008), a 484-page document that is largely text with some charts and photographs. Although it is a little more than a decade old, many of the current government publications cite research synthesized in this report. Furthermore, you can see in of August 2018 the Minister highlighted this report in her list of recommended resources. Published by the Public Health Agency of Canada, the assessment claims to provide "the most up-to-date synthesis of knowledge on how the health of Canadians is affected by the climate and what lies ahead under future climate scenarios" (2008, p. 4) As the authors speak to climate related health challenges of Canadians, and more particularly issues of vulnerability and adaptive capacity, there are definitive portions of this sizeable document that prove useful to my research. My focus was primarily on the first chapter *Climate Change and Health*, as it determines factors such approaches to studying climate change and health, who is at risk, vulnerabilities to impacts of climate change, adaptive capacity and a section titled "toward adaptation" (Public Health Agency of Canada, 2008, p. 3). For these reasons, this publication made for rich data to explore when paired with my research questions and theoretical framework.

I did not include the Federal Government Framework on Lyme disease listed in the Minister's letter as in general it did not relate to my research questions. I did review the other two items in her bullet points (specifically related to heat events and heat alerts) but including them would have been well beyond my resources and the scope of this project. Indeed, I had already gathered sufficient government documents that related generally to human health, vulnerability, persons with disabilities, and climate change in Canada.

As you can see in her closing paragraph, the Minister of Environment encouraged me to read the adaptation sections of Canada's 7th National Communication and 3rd Biennial Report and while it was not sufficient to use as data, some concepts helped to inform my analysis. In addition to this, I have included the last publication the Minister suggested, the *Working Group on Adaptation and Climate Resilience Final Report*. This report spans the federal, provincial, and territorial governments. It also informs the Pan-Canadian Framework, a framework that relies heavily on human adaptation to climate change. The Minister notes that these documents are part of a comprehensive look at adaptation and climate resilience across Canada. The *Adaptation and Climate Resilience Final Report* (2016b) I included as my sixth data source is a 53-page document that notably opens with reference (in French) to being available in French, but no options are given for other formats. Of particular interest to my study is the section on the importance of adaptation and climate resilience in Canada.

All six documents I have chosen as data provide comprehensive insights into the Canadian government's response to climate change in areas of human health. Following a thorough research process that included an official government correspondence, I felt confident that I was accessing the most relevant documents for my analysis. These six climate related publications are being used by individual Canadians as well as federal, provincial, and territorial governments and non-profit entities for resource and program planning. In these documents, government departments, scientists, and select industry partners offer their perspectives on what they call a synthesis of knowledge on climate change risks and the need for adaptation. As such, these six climate change documents are integral to individual climate change initiatives in Canada and their urgency, agency, and widespread use makes them excellent sources of data for this project.

Ethics

To help protect individuals and marginalized groups, it is essential to provide ethical safeguards within our research. I have collected data from publicly available Canadian government documents for this study and I have not used human participants. Early in my research phase, I contacted the University of Victoria's Human Research Ethics Department who confirmed that because my research does not utilize human participants or human biological materials, I did not need official approval. Nonetheless, I recognize that ethical matters extend far beyond what is categorized by an academic ethics system. Stacey Alaimo (2017), helps to illustrate my personal experience of ethics in saying that:

> While we might wish that all our ethical and political commitments would align and become so beautifully articulated as to be inseparable and synergistic, it is nonetheless often the case that historically rooted discursive and ideological formations mean that ethics, politics and scholarship take place within more messy, vexed, and contradictory terrains (p. ix).

In these ways, I acknowledge that my personal ethics extend far beyond what is categorized as ethics by an academic ethics system. Specifically, I reflect upon informed consent and confidentiality as I have used reflections acquired from individuals during my research gathering phase. I am careful to use vague and non-specific details when I write about the wide-ranging experiences of disability that I have been entrusted with. In addition, through my own self-reflexivity I identify my personal connections to this research, which at times has left me feeling quite vulnerable. It is a reflection of the ableism in our society that I fear disclosing too much about my own health struggles, specifically what these revelations could mean for my personal life, privacy, and career.

CHAPTER FOUR: Findings

This chapter synthesizes my analytical journey through six government documents introduced in the previous chapter. I expand upon my reflexive research process, tie together theoretical tenets presented in Chapters 2 and 3, and present interrelated themes and subthemes identified through my thematic analysis. In order to accomplish the latter, I include relevant quotes and extracts from the data to illustrate how health and disability are framed within six Canadian government climate change documents. As highlighted in my conceptual framework, a reflexive thematic analysis often follows a six-step process, while remaining flexible to researcher creativity. That is, the researcher's subjectivity is an analytic *resource* (Braun & Clarke, 2020). As a consequence of this personal method, my process of conducting poststructural, feminist, and critical disability-oriented research was a meaningful one. Over the last year, I revisited the data through the lens of my own health challenges, including a brain-injury. The personal experience of living with a differently abled body in a changing climate is necessarily political, as it is inextricably tied to societal structures and government policies. Meaning was derived since my data findings coalesced with my lived experience — a necessary component to any reflexive thematic analysis. As such, by following Braun and Clarke's (2006) flexible and immersive six-step process to thematic analysis, I was able to categorize pointed themes and subthemes that emerged from my careful readings of the data.

In the first part of this chapter, I bridge the conceptual tenets introduced in the previous chapter with the personal and adaptive methods used for my reflexive thematic analysis. That said, my examination of these documents is not designed to offer a singular, definitive *truth* about climate change and persons with disabilities. Canadian climate change strategies cannot present a singular truth about the reality of persons with disabilities; rather, the documents present a certain perspective, just as I do in my analysis.

With the above in mind, given that persons with disabilities (like other marginalized people) are more likely to be severely impacted by climate change than persons without disabilities, my most significant finding is the absence of disability perspectives from the climate strategy documents. Through careful reviews of the data set, I found that references to persons with disabilities and pre-existing health conditions were scarce, and I noted most significance in the stark absence of such perspectives. These Federal Government exclusions link to disability injustice, by allowing me to note where persons with disabilities could have been situated within the publications. This omission of non-normative bodies and minds is conceivably why the Minister of Environment and Climate Change rerouted my query about publications related to climate change and persons with disability, to a more general question about *vulnerable populations*. This is important term to interrogate, as Caria and Hayes (2019) note that when the phrase vulnerable groups is used as an umbrella term to signify underrepresented groups, it is never clear whose needs are being supported and whose skills are being utilized. Nonetheless, there remains a marked lack of attention paid to persons with disabilities in government climate change strategies, later in this chapter I point to the places where these considerations should appear, while uncovering embedded assumptions about health that explicitly appear.

Early on, I began to identify several codes and meanings in the climate change documents, including why and where certain relevant terms were used in each particular section. For instance, while coding, I mapped the occurrence of the term *vulnerability* by noting that while it often appeared in the documents, it was always poorly parsed by the authors. That is, who exactly is vulnerable and why they are vulnerable is not often considered in the climate change strategies. Indeed, vulnerable populations emerge in the data through embedded nods to anyone other than able-bodied, able-minded persons with the resources and capacities to adapt. Although I do not include this observation as a theme itself, like many other consequent findings, it is worth reporting for its relevance to disability justice.

Hegemonic notions of health and ability were embedded throughout all six of the documents I reviewed, while at the same time, the data set often contained contradictory and competing statements about health and climate change adaptation. Most documents, including the letter from Canada's Minister of Environment and Climate Change, touted adaptation as a primary pillar for climate change mitigation (for all persons, including vulnerable populations). Yet, buried within some of the documents, research was presented that showed adaptation has failed to be proven as an effective strategy to reduce climate harms. In fact, while the data set contained a few references to the intersecting and compounding struggles certain Canadians experience in their daily life, no connections were made in terms of how adaptation itself may increase these burdens. Coupled with a lack of evidence for the efficacy of climate change adaptation as a whole, there are many gaps in the strategies for persons with disabilities. Burdening already marginalized populations with more adaptation tasks, when these measures are not supported by evidence, is to further trouble their well-being. It is hard to know what to do with these specific findings; however, given that this is a poststructural inspired analysis, I simply point to the often messy, conflicting nature of the data. In this way, I conclude with these contradictions, not as a distinct theme but rather a curious finding from the data that is worth reporting.

Themes from the Data

A theme illustrates a significant occurrence within the data related to the research questions, and each theme speaks to patterns and meanings from the data set (Braun & Wilkinson, 2003; Braun & Clarke, 2006; Braun & Clarke, 2020). A theme is not always a quantifiable measure; rather, themes stem from what they capture in relation to the overall research question (Braun & Clarke, 2006; Braun & Clarke, 2020). In reflexive thematic analysis, themes are actively created by the researcher, through their own assumptions and interpretive frameworks (Braun, Clarke, & Hayfield, 2019). When I applied these guidelines for theme development alongside my conceptual framework (described in the previous chapter), three broad and compelling patterns emerged. Below, I list these core themes and subthemes, then subsequently provide extracts from the data to help illustrate each finding. I make note that their respective numbers are for reference only, and do not signify a weighted ranking of individual themes. More importantly, these three themes overlap and coalesce in ways I will review as I present a selection of quotes, lists, and figures from the six data sources. While I list my findings separately, it is integral to note that they are interlaced with one another, with common threads between all themes and subthemes.

1. Be *Adaptive* and *Resilient*. Subtheme: Adaptation to climate change is presented as both a central priority and an individual responsibility.

2. Healthy, normative bodies and minds are presumed. Subtheme: Individuals are generally understood as having the same capacity to adapt and a common ground for shared concerns.
3. Persons with disabilities are notably absent from the climate change documents. Subtheme: The economy is prioritized. Subtheme: Government climate change strategies are inaccessible to many people.

Be Adaptive and Resilient

The Canadian government presents resilience building and adaptation to climate change as critical priorities for individuals, governments, and private sectors. This theme is first illustrated in the titles of documents recommended to me by the Minister of Environment and Climate Change (McKenna, 2018): Expert Panel on Climate Change Adaptation and Resilience Results (2018); Sector Perspectives on Impacts and Adaptation (2014); Human Health in a Changing Climate; A Canadian Assessment of Vulnerabilities and Adaptive Capacity (2017); Adapting to Extreme Heat Events: Guidelines for Assessing Health Vulnerability (2011); Working Group on Adaptation and Climate Resilience Final Report (2019); as well as in the Minister's specific encouragement for me to read the adaptation sections of Canada's 7th National and 3rd Biennial Report (2018).

Moreover, the letter I received from Canada's Minister of Environment and Climate Change Catherine McKenna (2018) explicitly refers to *adaptation* and *resilience building* as key government directives for offsetting climatic threats. Demonstrating both adaptation and resilience as key government climate change priorities, I call attention to Figure 1, in which McKenna (2018) states that "Taking action to adapt to current and future climate change impacts is necessary to help protect Canadians from climate change risks, reduce costs and ensure that society remains resilient" (p. 2). Here, we see that the government conveys adaptation as essential (and necessary) in promoting individual resilience, economic growth, and protecting against climate hazards. Further, in the paragraph that follows the above quote, McKenna (2018) reports that the First Ministers of Canada adopted the Pan-Canadian Framework on Clean Growth and Climate Change including "adapt and build resilience" (p. 2) as one of its four foundational pillars for addressing climate change.

As the title suggests, Chapter 9 *Adaptation: Linking Research and Practice* is focused primarily on adaptation, with an emphasis on synthesizing research and recommendations for a number of adaptation activities (Eyzaguirre & Warren, 2014). Several obstacles are considered by the authors in this chapter, factors they suggest will help bridge the gaps between climate awareness and adaptive action. These government adaptation priorities include: building effective champions, strong leaders, and supportive policies (Eyzaguirre & Warren, 2014, p. 255). These terms are echoed across the data set but are never fully parsed. It remains unclear who the effective champions and strong leaders are and what diverse knowledge they bring to adaptation planning. Since the contributing authors in this chapter are from Health Canada, Ministries of the Environment, Ministry of Forest, Lands and Resources, Environment Canada, Natural Resources Canada, Ontario Centre for Climate Impacts and Adaptation, and the University of New Brunswick (from the Physical and Environmental Science Department) the reader is left to assume these leaders, champions, and policies stem from the same sectors. No other leaders or collaborators are listed as necessary or absent, and persons with disabilities are not referenced.

Section 4 of Chapter 7 is titled *Addressing Climate Change Risks to Health*, and here Berry et al. (2014) state that "adaptation is needed to reduce growing risks to vulnerable populations and communities" (p. 217). While it is clear that the government suggests adaptation is required to prepare for the impacts of climate change, a paragraph later on the same page seems to contradict the same suggestion. Berry et al. (2014) cite Lesnikowski et al. (2011) who state that information about the success of climate change adaptation efforts is limited. The latter point is not further investigated or considered in this chapter, but I include this statement as it shows where some themes from the data have curiously overlapped with contradictions in the same data source. I discuss this finding further in the conclusion of my analysis.

In Chapter 9, Eyzaguirre and Warren (2014) cite psychology research to explain why some people are reticent to adapt by quoting Gifford (2011) who states, "limitations in how we think, view the world and perceive risk figure prominently in the literature on psychological barriers to adaptation" (p. 273). Barriers here are framed as predominantly related to individual ways of thinking and viewing the world, as if individuals come to perceive risk from equal footing. Risk perception as it relates to the realities of living with disabilities (or from other marginalized positions) is not explored in the sections that speak to barriers to adaptation. The authors do not elaborate on why some groups may have more to contend with in the face of climate change but rather, Eyzaguirre and Warren (2014) instead repeat the notion that if some people were not limited in their ways of thinking about, viewing the world, and perceiving risk, they would be adequately prepared for climate change impacts.

Looking at the way risk perception is presented, it is clear that there are underlying assumptions and expectations in the documents, specifically in that each individual has equivalent access to both understanding and perceiving climate change threats and then acting to resist them with equal resources. This finding links back to the critique offered by Harvard Sociology Chair Jason Beckfield (2020), who states that adaptive action requires resources and a number of skills to mobilize these resources. These understandings relate directly to the taken-for-granted assumptions embedded in the previous extract, as how we think and perceive risk (and consequently act on that risk) is directly related to social inequities in our society.

Recognizing the harms of applying similar partial, mechanical approaches to these issues, many scholars note that deeper, more politicized climate change problems and solutions cannot be tended to in simplistic ways (Cameron, 2012; Mikulewicz, 2019). That is, climate change adaptation strategies are most frequently framed by governments as requiring techno-managerial solutions alone, rather than applying dynamic, social justice-based approaches. For example, in research that critiques the exclusion of colonialism from studies on Inuit vulnerability and adaptation in Canada, Cameron (2012) notes of the trouble in offering narrow solutions to climate:

> The vulnerability and adaptation literature re-frames the human dimensions of climatic change as something that can be assessed in community-based focus groups and targeted by specific, "local" policies. The deeply political origins of both climatic change and Inuit vulnerability to climatic change are rendered extraneous; they are simply not relevant to the question as it is posed. (p. 109)

The above quote helps to demonstrate how Canadian government climate change adaptation and resilience strategies are framed as both formulaic and apolitical, as evidenced by government strategies proposing problems be mitigated primarily through simple, individualized adaptive measures.

The *Adapting to Our Changing Climate in Canada* poster (Government of Canada, 2016a) opens with the title: *We have the knowledge to adapt now*! This quote illustrates a similar message: that the government has acquired the knowledge necessary, and that adaptation is a primary directive for combating climate change. The title is in large, bolded text and includes an exclamation point, suggesting urgency - that climate change knowledge is now held by the government and that immediate adaptive action is required. Here, the government emphasizes and hastens the urgency for a collective adapting to climate change without parsing who exactly is being asked to adapt and what varying obstacles they may have in adapting. In the paragraphs under the title, the authors share that further climate change is inevitable and that we must reduce greenhouse gas emissions to limit climate change: "Therefore adaptation is also critical" (Government of Canada Poster, 2016a).

In the Public Health Agency of Canada's publication, *Climate Change Impacts on the Health of Canadians* (2007), the authors claim that "as the climate continues to change and impacts on health are increasingly evident, adaptation is needed to reduce growing risks to vulnerable populations and communities" (p. 11). Here, adaptation is cited as a necessary response to climate threats, specifically within vulnerable groups. While it is evident that adaptation is presented by the government as a primary pillar to protect against climate change, the authors do not follow with disability specific limits, challenges, or supports to adaptation for persons with disabilities. Furthermore, persons with disabilities are not listed or specified within the categorization of vulnerable groups.

Climate Disasters

One of the main textual sources of information in the poster (Figure 2) is highlighted in large font as *Adapting – There's a lot we can do!* (Government of Canada, 2016a). As seen within the previous quote, the use of the personal plural pronoun *we* is found in several places on the poster, yet there is no explanation related to *we* are and what *we* can or cannot do. Below the *we* message on this publication is a short list of information that relates to what individuals can do, particularly in response to climate and weather-related emergencies. While the poster suggests there is *a lot* that can be done to prepare for climate events, the list is short and lacks specific, descriptive, and informative measures. The heading *Adapting – There's a lot we can do!* then follows with the directive of *There's a lot you can do* (Government of Canada, 2016a). I notice here how the message narrows from a shared *we* perspective to an individualized *you* directive.

Underneath a section of the poster that suggests there is a lot *you* can do to adapt to climate change is a section that reads, "There are many things you can do to reduce your risk from a changing climate, such as listening for heat alerts and storm warnings and being prepared for extreme events by creating an emergency kit" (Government of Canada, 2016a). Here, we see the government placing responsibility for adapting to climate change onto individuals, specifically when asking them to create an emergency kit. Partnerships, lists, or other supports for creating these kits are not listed.

In the section of the poster that follows the title *Adapting, there's a lot we can do,* there are three adaptive suggestions offered: listening for heat alerts, listening for storm warnings, and preparing an emergency kit (Government of Canada, 2018). Here, I identified themes of adaptation and resilience building interlocking with the subtheme of individualized responsibility. Suggestions such as listening for heat/storm warnings and creating emergency kits are an example of problematizing and simplifying select issues and then placing the responsibility on individuals to adapt to the threats. The poster does not provide individuals, social workers, caregivers, and other allied health professionals strategies for the emergency kits to be prepared and funded for persons with disabilities and/or financially insecure communities. Through my own research, I did find the Federal Government provides a list of emergency essentials in a separate online *Emergency Preparedness Guide* for *People with Disabilities/Special Needs* (getprepared.gc.ca). The emergency checklist and related webpage information is based on a government publication that is cited as being a co-operative effort between public and private organizations, consulted for their expertise and special insights. In order to showcase what is suggested for basic emergency kits, the list below is extracted from the Government of Canada's (2018) Emergency Preparedness Guide for People with Disabilities/Special Needs:

Basic emergency kit checklist:

- *Water* — two litres of water per person per day (include small bottles)
- *Food* that won't spoil, such as canned food, energy bars and dried foods (replace once a year)
- *Manual can opener*
- *Wind-up or battery-powered flashlight* (and extra batteries)
- *Wind-up or battery-powered radio* (and extra batteries)

- *First aid kit*
- *Special items such as prescription medications; Medic Alert bracelet; identification*
- *Extra keys* for your car and house
- *Cash, in smaller bills, such as $10 bills* and change for payphones
- *Special items according to your needs (i.e., prescription medication, infant formula, special equipment, pet food and water)*
- A copy of your emergency plan and contact information
- Other: ___________________________

Recommended additional items checklist:

- Two additional litres of water per person per day for cooking and cleaning
- Candles and matches or lighter (place in sturdy containers and do not burn unattended)
- Change of clothing and footwear for each household member
- Sleeping bag or warm blanket for each household member
- Toiletries, hand sanitizer, utensils
- Garbage bags for personal sanitation
- Toilet paper
- Minimum a week's supply of prescription medication
- Household chlorine bleach or water purifying tablets
- Basic tools (hammer, pliers, wrench, screwdrivers, work gloves, dust mask, knife)
- Small fuel-operated stove and fuel
- Whistle (in case you need to call for help)
- Duct tape (i.e., to tape up windows, doors, air vents)

- Detailed list of all special needs items, in the event they need to be replaced

I include these substantial lists as emergency kits are listed as part of climate adaptation in the government poster, and other strategy documents. While emergency kits are suggested throughout the climate adaptation strategies, I note that the challenges many people face in preparing and sustaining these supplies are not addressed. At the same time, in Chapter 7, *Human Health* by Berry et al. (2014), within a lengthy paragraph focused on increased research on impacts, education and the benefits of preparedness, Berry et al. (2014) note the need for "addressing root causes that limit preparedness e.g. poverty" (p. 217). Yet, in the public messages, such as the Government of Canada (2016a) adaptation poster, these realities are missing.

The Adaptation Process

The following figure from Chapter 7, *Human Health*, illustrates the government's broad emphasis on adaptation. In this section of the chapter, Berry et al. (2014) outline a seven-step adaptation process. The paragraph that proceeds the figure reads: "Governments, often on a partnered basis, have implemented a range of initiatives to understand how adaptation occurs among different groups and to encourage further action" (Berry, et al., 2014, p. 260).

Figure 3

Seven Steps Depicting the Adaptation Process

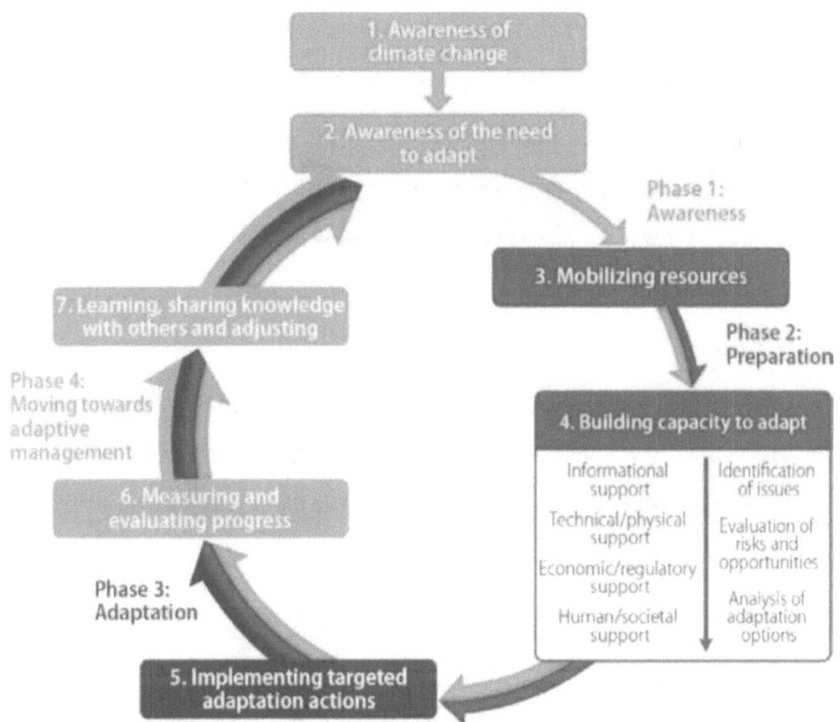

[IMAGE DESCRIPTION: The seven steps of the adaptation process are presented as a counter-clockwise cycle connected by blue, red, purple, and green arrows with corresponding coloured text boxes for each step.]

Note. The above figure is presented in a box captioned with bold letters stating: **THE ADAPTATION PROCESS** and includes and a detailed commentary for each step (Berry, Clarke, Fleury & Parker, 2014, p. 260).

The authors define the seven steps of the adaptation process in a corresponding list to the left of the cyclical figure. Adaptation is again presented as a principal solution to the effects of climate change. Here, in *step two*, the theme of adaptation as a requirement is explicitly conferred: awareness of the need to adapt. I point to another major theme that appears in this process: the absence of disability from each of the seven stages of the adaptation process.

As shown in Figure 3, *awareness of the need to adapt* is the second step in the adaptation process and as the authors state, "an awareness of the magnitude of the problem helps to identify adaptation as solution" (Berry et al., 2014, p. 260). Adaptation is again presented as a primary solution to climate change.

The adaptation messages conveyed in this section also link to other themes and subthemes in my analysis, such as the exclusion of persons with disabilities and the assumption that everyone has a uniform ability to adapt. In the large text commentary presented below Figure 4, the authors explain how certain groups already have an awareness of climate change, yet who these groups are is not established. Awareness of the need to adapt then follows with the message that several local and federal government groups boast adaptation programs and initiatives (Berry et al., 2014). Here, I observe how the government frames climate change as a techno-managerial problem while offering an over-simplified seven-step adaptation solution. Persons with disabilities (or vulnerable populations), and their various biological and social constraints to adaptation are not mentioned.

In summary, adaptation is presented as a fundamental climate change mitigation strategy, while attention to adaptation processes and challenges specific to persons with disabilities are absent. Adger (2009) reminds us that "adaptation to climate change, and hence the limits to adaptation, can only be understood in context" (p. 340). While adaptation directives are taken up by government authorities in the documents, contextual limits to adaptation for persons with disabilities are not examined.

Presuming Healthy, Normative Bodies and Minds

In the Government of Canada (2016a) poster, the authors state that this poster is a "useful adaptation tool for educators, private sectors, NGOs, etc.". The information that follows is from the one section on the poster that speaks specifically to protecting human health from extreme heat:

> *Protecting Canadian health from extreme heat.* With climate change the number of extreme weather events like heat waves is expected to increase. Many Canadian communities are already experiencing a greater number of hot days. Extreme heat can impact health, causing illness and even death.

Healthy bodies and minds without disease are embedded as the normative state of individuals targeted by these statements. Notable in this extract is a phrase that cites extreme heat from climate change as the element *causing* illness. Chronic disease and disabilities often commix with extreme heat in calamitous ways, yet these realities are absent here.

Illustrating a similar absence of disability and embedded baseline health, the following table is found in *Sector Perspectives on Impacts and Adaptation* by Berry and Clarke (2014). This list is adapted from the Seguin (2008) document, both included in my data sources. Here, Berry and Clarke (2014) summarize the same *key health concerns* from climate change that are echoed across the data set:

1. Heat-related illnesses and deaths
2. Respiratory and cardiovascular disorders
3. Possible changed patterns of illness and death due to cold
4. Death, injury and illness from violent storms, floods, etc.
5. Psychological health effects, including mental health and stress-related illnesses
6. Health impacts due to food or water shortages
7. Illnesses related to drinking water contamination
8. Effects of the displacement of populations and crowding in emergency shelters
9. Indirect health impacts from ecological changes, infrastructure damages and interruptions in health services
10. Eye, nose and throat irritation, and shortness of breath
11. Exacerbation of respiratory conditions
12. Chronic obstructive pulmonary disease and asthma
13. Exacerbation of allergies
14. Increased risk of cardiovascular diseases (heart attacks and ischemic heart disease)
15. Premature death
16. Sporadic cases and outbreaks of disease from strains of water-borne pathogenic micro-organisms
17. Food-borne illnesses
18. Other diarrheal and intestinal diseases
19. Impacts on nutrition due to availability of local and traditional foods
20. Increased incidence of vector-borne infectious diseases native to Canada (eastern and western equine encephalitis, Rocky Mountain spotted fever)

21. Introduction of infectious diseases new to Canada
22. Possible emergence of new diseases, and re-emergence of those previously eradicated in Canada
23. More cases of sunburns, skin cancers, cataracts and eye damage
24. Various immune disorders (p. 195)

I have purposefully extracted this lengthy list of health concerns as it helps to visually convey the negligible inclusion of any pre-existing health conditions. Most of the lines on this 24-point list highlight several health conditions each, yet there is only nominal mention of persons who already contend with physical, intellectual, psychiatric, or other disabilities in the face of climate change. In fact, the only pre-existing *health concerns* included are:

11. Exacerbation of respiratory conditions
13. Exacerbation of allergies

In this summary of key health considerations from climate change, the authors use the term "exacerbation" (Berry & Clarke, p. 195) when referring only to respiratory conditions and allergies. There are only two points that speak to any prior illness, obscured within a large table of *key health concerns*. Persons with disabilities do not appear.

Mental Health

On the Government of Canada (2017) website, under a section titled *mental health and wellness*, the government shares that one in three Canadians will experience mental illness in their lifetime. Yet, along with the above examples of a normalized body, there is a healthy mind assumed in the climate documents. This is evidenced by psychological and mental health effects stated only as *projected* concerns while any pre-existing mental health conditions are absent. Within the key health concerns listed above, item 5 is *psychological health effects from climate change and climate related events* (Berry & Clarke, 2014). The authors do not include the *exacerbation* of existing psychiatric or mental illness in the list of key health concerns from climate change. There is a marked absence of those who live with pre-existing psychological health challenges and stress-related illnesses.

In Chapter 7, *Human Health*, Berry et al. (2014) discuss "PSYCHOSOCIAL AND MENTAL HEALTH IMPACTS" (p. 208) related to climate change. The authors refer to a previous government publication by Berry et. al (2008) in which the authors state that:

> Symptoms of psychosocial impacts from an extreme weather event or disaster may take various forms such as alterations in mood, thoughts, behaviour, an increased level of distress, and a reduction of one's ability to function in everyday life. (p. 280)

Berry et al. (2014) also state:

> Disaster-induced cognitive and emotional issues may manifest in the form of concentration and memory loss, learning disorders, anxiety, acute stress disorders, PTSD, depression, sleep difficulties, aggression, substance abuse, and high-risk behaviour in adolescents. (p. 280)

Not only are acute stress disorders prioritized in this document, a *causal* relationship between disaster-induced mental health concerns and climate change is underscored. Referring to a figure in their chapter, Berry et al. (2014) state that there are causal pathways by which climate change affects mental health (p. 280). I do not dispute the connection between climate change and mental health, yet I point to how climate change is only presented as the *cause* of health concerns and mental health conditions, and the people who already contend with psychiatric health challenges in the face of climate change are absent.

In their report on mental health in a changing climate, Clayton et al. (2017) cite an ever-growing body of research demonstrating that those with pre-existing mental health challenges have increased sensitivity to the changing climate. Furthermore, Clayton et al. (2017) list comorbid mental health impacts from climate change, which include increased substance abuse, depression, anxiety, trauma, shock, and sleep disorders. Similarly, Anderson, Ziedonis, and Najavits (2014) found that compared with non-disabled groups, persons with physical disabilities experience more lifetime trauma and post-traumatic stress disorder (PTSD). These realities are absent from the health concerns listed across my data set.

Where are Persons with Disabilities?

While coding the data through my reflexive thematic analysis process, I noticed through straightforward searches that references related to persons with disabilities were absent from most of the documents. Specifically, the words *disability* and *disabilities* are widely missing from the climate change strategy conversations. For example, in the document *Adapting to Extreme Heat Events: Guidelines for Assessing Health Vulnerability* (2011), the words disability and disabilities do not appear. Similarly, in Chapter 7 (Berry et al., 2014), a chapter specifically titled *Human Health*, the terms disability and disabilities are not found. Likewise, in *Human Health in a Changing Climate: A Canadian Assessment of Vulnerabilities and Adaptive Capacity* (Seguin, 2008) the word *disabilities* does not appear, while the word *disability* is only found once across 484 pages. In this one occurrence, the reference is specific to a section on seniors, where the author notes:

> Compared with other adult populations, seniors are often more vulnerable because increasing age is highly correlated with increasing illness, disability, medication use and reduced fitness. (p. 71)

Certainly, disability exists in non-senior populations, yet this reality is missing from the extensive report. As such, the theme of persons with disabilities being absent from the climate change strategies is truly best relayed as it exists, by omission.

The following figure from the *Working Group on Adaptation and Climate Resilience Final Report*, Government of Canada (2016b) demonstrates a more nuanced absence of disability perspectives in the data. As stated in the letter from the Minister of Environment and Climate Change (2018), this report is said to "provide a comprehensive picture of adaptation and climate resilience actions being implemented across Canada" (p. 2).

Figure 4

The Ways in Which Climate Change Affects Health and Well-Being

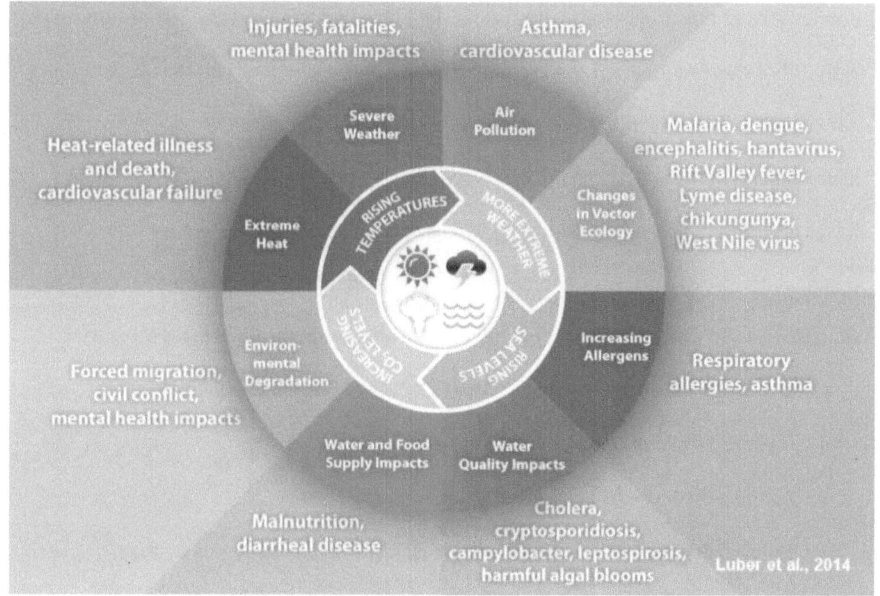

[IMAGE DESCRIPTION: Three concentric circles depict climate change related weather and environmental events. The centre circle features a red sun, a black cloud with a green lightning bolt, blue waves, and a white tornado cloud. Beyond the circles the eight outermost categories provide information on the health effects of climate change.]

Note. The above figure is taken from the *Working Group on Adaptation and Climate Resilience Final Report* (2016b, p. 8) and is found under the section heading *1.1.6. Health and Well-Being.*

This extract is from one of the more recent documents recommended to me by the Minister of Environment and Climate Change (in my response to my questions about publications related to persons with disabilities). The figure is used as a visual summary alongside a short four paragraph section on *Health and Well-Being*, and the illustration is not explained by the text that surrounds it, except for the title: *Overview of the ways in which climate change affects health and well-being* (Government of Canada, 2016b). An image description was not provided. As you can see, climactic events and weather i.e., rising sea level, extreme temperatures, water, and food impacts are depicted in the three centre circles. In this Government of Canada (2016b) figure, the outermost categories describe the following ways in which climate change affects health and well-being:

- Injuries, fatalities, mental health impacts,
- Asthma, cardiovascular disease
- Malaria, dengue, encephalitis, hantavirus, Rift Valley fever, Lyme disease, chikungunya, West Nile virus
- Respiratory allergies, asthma
- Cholera, cryptosporidiosis, campylobacter, leptospirosis, harmful algal blooms
- Malnutrition, diarrheal disease
- Forced migration, civil conflicts, mental health impacts
- Heat-related illness and death, cardiovascular failure (p. 8)

This government document describes this figure as providing a comprehensive overview of the ways in which climate change impacts health and well-being, yet as I have done with other examples from the data, I point to not just what is included, but who and what is left out. I do not dispute the need for awareness of the increasing emergence of these health conditions, rather, I call attention to the absence of pre-existing disease, disability, and impacts related to the exacerbation of chronic, comorbid conditions, including mental illness. In this list, climate change impacts on health and well-being are only considered for normative bodies and minds without pre-existing disease. A standard, healthy body-mind is the embedded suggestion in the above list. Moreover, visually impaired individuals are excluded by the absence of image descriptions and text-based explanations for this figure. Looking to the poster *Adapting to Our Changing Climate in Canada – We have the knowledge to adapt now!* (Government of Canada, 2016a), there is an assumption of a normalized, healthy Canadian. Specifically, I call attention to the associated photographs and human figure depictions in this poster extract.

Figure 5

Adapting to our Changing Climate in Canada (a)

WEATHER ALERT
Adapting –
There's a lot we can do!
There are many things that you can do to reduce your risks from a changing climate, such as listening for heat alerts and storm warnings and being prepared for extreme events by creating an emergency kit.
Teachers: Check out Climate Change Lessons at ontarioecoschools.org and cobwebsim.com.

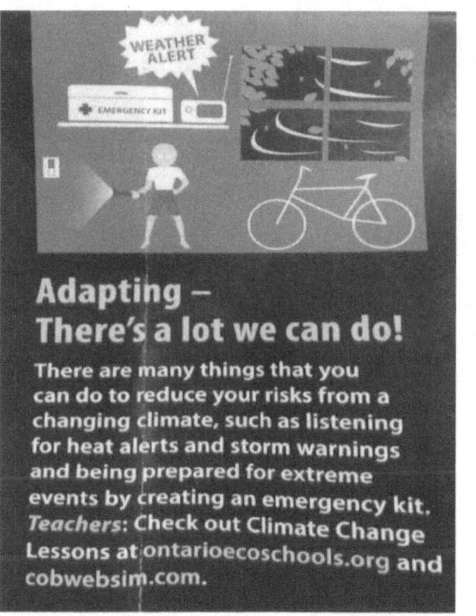

[IMAGE DESCRIPTION: A standing white cartoon figure holds a flashlight, surrounded by a bicycle, a shelf with an emergency kit, radio and weather alert text box and a window with blowing wind and snow.]

Note. Excerpt from the poster Adapting to our Changing Climate in Canada (Government of Canada, 2016a).

The addition of a bicycle (shown in figure 5) speaks to assumed abilities to both own and ride a bicycle while simultaneously delivering a message about individual responsibilities to cycle (in an effort to personally reduce greenhouse gas emissions). Commenting on similar themes within social policy strategies, Brodie (2007) notes that concepts of individualization are designed to shape citizens into autonomous market actors while obscuring a notion of choice. Here, the government poster conveys implicit assumptions about both accessibility and responsibility, while lacking more diverse and just perspectives and depictions.

Figure 6

Adapting to our Changing Climate in Canada (b)

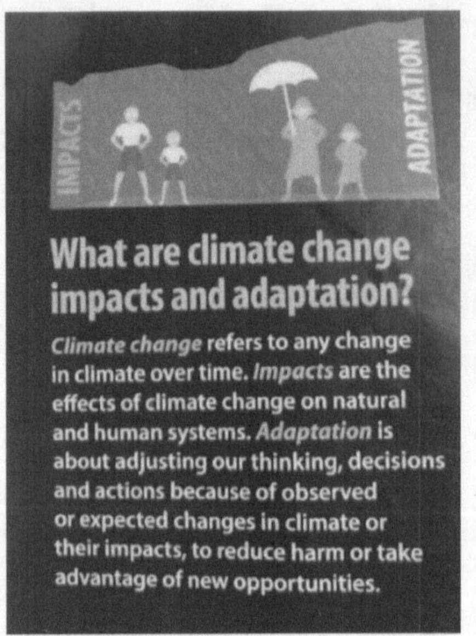

[IMAGE DESCRIPTION: Four white cartoon figures are standing in the rain, two adults and 2 children. One adult is holding an umbrella. The words IMPACTS and ADAPTATION are positioned vertically in upper case on either side.]

Note. Excerpt from the poster Adapting to our Changing Climate in Canada (Government of Canada, 2016a).

Through my process detailing image descriptions, I was able to examine nuanced representations of Canadians. For example, a total of five cartoon human figures accompany the information in the poster (see Figures 5 and 6) which include short sections of texts that speak to climate impacts, adaptation, and personal responsibility. All five humans are white, and all of the figures are standing. One is carrying an umbrella in the rain while one is holding a flashlight. Persons with disabilities are absent from the text of this document and light-skinned, able-bodies are depicted by the figures.

In addition to the above excerpt, the right side of the Government of Canada (2016a) poster includes photographs of four individuals (all appear to be men) and each are in productive, action-oriented positions, from walking to taking notes on a work site, to standing and assessing sea level rise, and one is laying on the ice measuring sea level thickness. The men presented in the poster appear able-bodied and are engaged in productive work activities.

Another example within the theme of excluding persons with disabilities from climate adaptation strategies is found in the following extract from Chapter 9. Highlighting the *Barriers and Limitations to Adaptation*, Eyzaguirre and Warren state (2014):

> This section expands on barriers and challenges to adaptation identified in Chapters 3 to 8 of this Assessment. It considers the role of information and communications, resources, governance and norms, psychology and values, and leadership in hindering progress on adaptation by various stakeholder groups. (p. 269)

This section emerges as an important example for illustrating the absence and exclusion of persons with disabilities in Canadian climate change adaptation strategies. The authors state that the barriers and challenges to adaptation are synthesized from six full chapters (3-8) of the larger assessment. Who constitutes *various stakeholder groups* is not identified. The table and surrounding text (summarizing barriers and limitations to adaptation) do not list persons with disabilities as stakeholders, and there is no reference to the unique climate adaptation barriers and challenge varied groups may experience. Below, types of barriers and challenges to adaptation are summarized in five categories: information and communication; resources (economics, skills, technology); governance and norms; psychology; and values and leadership, with examples given for each (Eyzaguirre & Warren, 2014).

Figure 7

Barriers and Challenges to Adaptation

Type of barrier / challenge	Example	Chapter
Information and communications	Difficulties teasing out multiple influences on visitation choices (e.g. fuel price, transportation costs, border restrictions, reputation, demographic and market trends) from climate change impacts	5
	Mismatch between spatial and temporal resolution of climate projections and management needs. Difficulties obtaining reliable projections at scales relevant to management needs	3, 5, 6
	Availability of guidance to interpret climate scenarios and factor modeling outputs into infrastructure and mine closure design	3
	Lack of data and information on weather extremes (e.g. future patterns of rainfall extremes)	5, 8
	Limited data and information on past and future sector-specific climate change impacts (e.g. climate change impacts on forests, wind, solar and biomass energy production; water-related impacts of climate change and implications for oil sands development, shale gas and enhanced oil recovery; climate change impacts on water resource infrastructure, health impacts)	3, 7, 8
Resources (economic, skills, technology)	Few incentives for action beyond business as usual (e.g. incremental cost of applying existing engineering or technological solutions to adapt mine operations to climate change, or of preserving ecological goods and services on agricultural lands)	3, 5, 6
	Lack of expertise and understanding surrounding local impacts of climate change on business operations, and effective adaptation solutions	5
	Limited adaptation options for snowmobiling (e.g. widespread implementation of snowmaking is impractical)	5
	Lack of financial resources for surveillance, prevention and control of vector-borne diseases; expertise and capacity to diagnose emerging vector-borne diseases, licensed and effective products for disease-vector control	7
Governance and norms	Complexities redefining sustainable forest management related to number of players and trade-offs involved	3
	Influence of non-climate stressors, such as region-wide demographic changes and rural outmigration	4
	Reliable access to non-commercial food supplies at risk if infrastructure integrity is vulnerable to climate change	4
	Designs based on future climate projections shift paradigm from building code and current design approaches	5
	Coastal adaptation plans typically led by government agencies outside of public health such that health impacts may not considered	7
Psychology and values	Perceived importance of climate change low relative to economic challenges, job losses and mill closures facing the sector	3
	Uncertainty in future climate change projections hinders investment decisions on adaptation	3
	Optimism about capacity to overcome climate change adaptation challenges	5
	Continued focus on replacement of aging infrastructure, on capacity upgrades to deal with increasing population and on changing regulatory requirements to address risks to water supply infrastructure – with the role of changing codes, standards and related instruments receiving less attention	8
Leadership	Proactive adaptation planning in mining is rare despite use of climate scenarios for impact assessment and identification of monitoring and adaptation strategies	3
	Taking a 'wait-and-see approach' due to difficulties finding the correct balance between waiting for more information to inform future action and taking action in the short term based on available information	3

TABLE 4: Barriers and challenges to adaptation highlighted in previous chapters

[IMAGE DESCRIPTION: Five categories of *barriers and challenges to adaptation* are presented by the authors in a blue and white table, with examples given for each.]

Note. Reproduced from "Barriers and challenges to adaptation highlighted in previous chapters" by Eyzaguirre and Warren (2014, p. 270).

Here, I point to who and what is absent from the table. For instance, under the barrier/challenge listed as *Resources (economic, skills, technology*) Eyzaguirre and Warren (2014) provide the following examples:

- Few incentives for action beyond business as usual (incremental cost of applying existing engineering or technological solutions to adapt mine operations to climate change, or of preserving ecological goods and services on agricultural lands)
- Lack of expertise and understanding surrounding local impacts of climate change on business operations, and effective adaptation solutions
- Limited adaptation options for snowmobiling (widespread implementation of snowmaking is impractical)
- Lack of financial resources for surveillance, prevention and control of vector-borne diseases; expertise and capacity to diagnose emerging vector-borne diseases; licensed and effective products for disease-vector control (p. 270)

Climate change resource barriers and challenges felt by persons with disabilities and other marginalized populations are notably absent from this list and the broader table.

At the same time, four of the five summarized categories focus markedly on industry (such as mining, oil sands, and oil recovery), with one of the five categories speaking to particular human health factors. Within this category of psychology and values, persons with disabilities and pre-existing mental health/medical conditions are missing. Rather, there is a marked emphasis on economic challenges in this category. The segment in this chapter pertaining to "perceived importance of climate change low relative to economic challenges and job losses and mill closures facing the sector" (Eyzaguirre & Warren, 2014, p. 270) is the most considered by the authors.

Persons with disabilities and vulnerable populations are not listed as stakeholders in Chapter 9, *Adaptation: Linking Research and Practice* (Eyzaguirre & Warren, 2014). As seen in the table above, economic threats are highlighted, yet they are hinged to employment and industry. Where the authors demonstrate the limitations of adaptation based on financial barriers, they state the most significant barriers to climate change will be felt by businesses, and provincial and municipal governments (Eyzaguirre & Warren, 2014). That is, the financial constraints related to climate change are overwhelmingly cited as matters of employment and government. In summary, personal responsibility to climate change adaptation is assumed and expected, and I observe government fiscal priorities taking precedence.

Prioritizing Economy

In the document *Human Health in a Changing Climate: A Canadian Assessment of Vulnerabilities and Adaptive Capacity* (Séguin, 2008), the consistent theme of taken-for-granted assumption of baseline productive body-mind is linked to economy:

> Climate change can also have an impact through economic and social factors such as the loss of employment or property after a natural disaster, resulting in stress and other illnesses. Climate change will also exacerbate the challenges already faced by many Canadian communities that rely on agriculture, forestry and other natural resource-based activities. (p. 13)

In the first sentence above, the authors refer to economic and social impacts of climate change. Loss of employment and property damage are the examples provided that *result* in stress and other illnesses.

The second half of the first sentence includes the claim that climate change impacts result in stress and other illnesses, i.e., the consequences of losing one's job and property is listed as the cause that then *results* in stress and other illnesses (Séguin, 2008). Stress and other illnesses are presented in the documents as being the *result* of job loss and loss of property, and people who live with prior disease are missing. Moreover, this economy heavy focus is in a section specific to issues related to *climate change and human health*, yet the discussion fails to consider climate change health effects on persons with disabilities. This finding is akin to what Goodley (2014) describes as *neoliberal-ableism*, a strategy that esteems both this normalized body-mind, and abled citizens who are economically prolific and dependant on neoliberal systems of capitalist production.

Chapter 9, *Adaptation: Linking Research and Practice* (Eyzaguirre & Warren, 2014) further demonstrates the Federal Government's fiscal priority in adaptation to climate change. Figure 3 in this chapter includes two pie charts that demonstrate the federal government's fiscal "evolution" (Eyzaguirre & Warren, 2014, p. 263). These pie charts illustrate a five-year trend toward more of an economic investment in adaptation programs. This section appears to be a defense to criticism on the lack of accountable leadership toward adaptation, as the rhetoric clearly illuminates the economic priorities of the government. Figure 3 on p. 270 of the Eyzaguirre and Warren (2014) chapter *Adaptation: Linking Research and Practice*, lists barriers to adaptation that are also relevant to the government's prioritizing of economy. This table summarizes data from the six previous chapters and lists them within five barrier categories. Within each barrier, examples are listed for each: market trends, management needs, infrastructure, mine closures, biomass energy production, oil sands development, shale gas, enhanced oil recovery, business, engineering, technological solutions, business operations, sustainable forest management, economic challenges, job losses, and mill closures (Eyzaguirre & Warren, 2014, p. 270). I do not dispute the importance of many of these examples for the wellbeing and livelihood of Canadians, rather I point to the theme of prioritizing economy while simultaneously excluding persons with disabilities from these conversations.

The Inaccessibility of Government Climate Change Strategies

Another subtheme that emerged within the category of exclusion is inaccessibility. In keeping with quality practice in reflexive thematic analysis, it is important for me to again situate myself here. Specifically, I note that I explored these adaptation strategies not only as a social work researcher, but also as a person with disabilities concerned about climate related impacts on my own health. Through my close review of the selected government texts and images, I found many similar examples of exclusionary practices and ways in which the information was presented within a broader context of inaccessibility. To this point, I could not read the Government of Canada (2016a) poster when I found it online, only the italicized tagline that states: *Together, we have the knowledge to adapt now.* The web version and English text was small and blurry (see https://www.nrcan.gc.ca/sites/www.nrcan.gc.ca/files/earthsciences/images/assess/2016/adaptation_poster_e.jpg). There is an option to print the poster, yet many persons with disabilities, and those with limited incomes, do not have a printer at home. Through my research I discovered individuals can fill out an on-line form or call 1-800-387-2000 to request up to two posters in English or French to be sent to your home free of charge (product # M174-13/2016). I was able to use the on-line order form and within two weeks the full-colour 24" by 36" poster was sent to me. It was only then that I could read the information on this poster. Further highlighting accessibility challenges, a friend who lives with disabilities wanted to view this poster and she underscored the importance of having image descriptions so as to make photos and other visual imagery accessible to people who are visually impaired (as assistive technologies can read and describe the images to them). Image descriptions were not included for any of the Canadian government climate change publications I reviewed, including this poster. The government claims this poster contains *accessible* climate change information for "educators, community groups, NGOs" (Government of Canada, 2016a). Having said that, individuals who are visually impaired, those with low literacy, who lack computer and internet access, and who speak languages other than English and French will have trouble accessing this information. In addition, I have not seen this poster in any community space, medical office, or government building.

In Chapter 9, *Adaptation: Linking Research and Practice*, the authors state that workshops are frequently used as tools to raise climate awareness and stimulate local adaptation (Eyzaguirre & Warren, 2014). Section 5 is titled *Overcoming Barriers and Facilitating Action* and Ezyaguirre and Warren (2014) note "the first step towards adaptation implementation is awareness of climate change, potential impacts and the need to adapt" (p. 274). Further, Eyzaguirre and Warren (2014) state:

> Workshops are frequently used as a mechanism to raise awareness and stimulate local adaptation. These typically bring together people with expertise in climate change science and adaptation with community leaders, municipal staff and *sometimes* the general public. (p. 274)

I question who is represented *sometimes* in these workshops, and while I endeavoured to find out the general demographics of those who attended these events, this information is not made available.

Missing from this section on *overcoming barriers* is the reality that childcare, mobility, costs, and general accessibility come into play when considering workshop attendance for many people (including persons with disabilities). Linking environmental justice and social work practice, Erickson (2018) notes that most groups affected by environmental injustices do not have the privileges required to get involved with related policy work and thus these voices are underrepresented. As it is not made clear by the government publications, I question how workshop attendees are selected and if there is a process in place to ensure a wide representation. Persons with disabilities are not cited.

Chapter 9 (Eyzaguirre & Warren, 2014) contains numerous health data-visualization tools, interactive visuals, maps, and other graphics to portray scientific data on climate impacts. As the research presented by the government is offered in English text (and sometimes French), many persons with visual, cognitive, and other impairments, as well as language needs, would not be able to access these climate data-visualization tools. In Chapter 9, Eyzaguirre and Warren (2014) claim that interactive graphics are excellent tools to stimulate discussion on climate awareness, yet this media is prohibitive to many people.

Relatedly, Chapter 7, *Human Health* (Berry et al., 2014) is found within the larger document *Canada in a Changing Climate: Sector Perspectives on Impacts and Adaptation*. In this chapter, the government specifically addresses human health and vulnerable populations. This publication is only available in English (as a PDF on the Government of

Canada's Natural Resources website). The 41-page document is introduced as being led by Natural Resources Canada, with the involvement of over 90 authors and 115 expert reviewers and is said to have been a synthesis of over 1500 recent publications (Government of Canada, 2019). The authors are employees of Health Canada and the Public Health Agency of Canada, and the chapter includes contributions from authors associated with Environment Canada, Health Canada, Public Health Agency of Canada, Centre for Coastal Health, and one Environmental Consultant (an energy policy researcher). This 41-page, full colour, PDF chapter is divided into 7 sections including key findings and references: including tables, figures, boxes, and case studies with English text. Coupled with the English (only) text, there are no descriptive images.

As well as the more practical and overt findings of inaccessibility, I searched the data set for the word accessibility and what is being said at each finding. For example, in Chapter 7 on *Human Health* by Berry et al. (2014) accessibility is mentioned twice. One instance is in a table related to "urban and rural characteristics that increase vulnerability to climate change and climate-related impacts" (Berry et al., 2014, p. 215). Here, Berry et al. (2014) list one of the vulnerability factors as "Limited availability and accessibility of public services and programs and communication venues to deliver health and emergency messages" (p. 215). I list this occurrence as it links both to the subtheme of inaccessibility as well as contradictions in the data. While the strategies note an awareness of the need for programs and communications to be *accessible*, what this accessibility means in practical terms is missing from the data.

Relatedly, I searched Chapter 9, *Adaptation: Linking Research and Practice* (Eyzaguirre & Warren, 2014) for the term accessibility. In this 33-page chapter the term *accessibility* is mentioned once, while the terms inaccessible and inaccessibility do not appear. Where barriers and challenges to adaptation are presented (see Figure 7) Eyzaguirre and Warren (2014) state:

> Barriers and challenges related to information for adaptation continue to be widely-cited as factors constraining action in Canada. Previous chapters in this assessment highlight issues related to the availability and accessibility of data and information on both average and extreme climate conditions, climate projections and their interpretation, climate change impacts research, and methods and tools to help integrate climate change information into decision making. (p. 270)

This extract illustrates how accessibility in these documents is hinged to access of climate conditions and research related to climate impacts and decision-making; rather than a consideration for auditory, visual, motor, mobility, cognitive and other access challenges.

Comparably, the term *accessible* appears in the *Adaptation: Linking Research and Practice* chapter (Eyzaguirre & Warren, 2014) three times. The context is consistent with the above example in that accessible/accessibility is not linked to persons with disabilities. For example, in a section specific to *Overcoming Barriers* to adaptation, Eyzaguirre and Warren (2014) report that:

> Decision makers are looking for the right type of information, at an appropriate scale and level of detail that is accessible and understandable. Over the past 5 years there has been an increase in the availability and quality of climate scenarios. Several groups in Canada have focused on providing scenario data, and making it publicly accessible (the Canadian Climate Change Scenarios Network, the Pacific Climate Impacts Consortium, and Ouranos). These groups assist decision makers in

> adapting to climate change by providing access to relevant and useable data, maps and graphs of future climate conditions. (p. 276)

Above, the term accessible is referenced twice unrelated to persons with disabilities. The third and final time the word accessible appears in this chapter relates to previous versions of adaptation assessments, where Eyzaguirre and Warren (2014) state:

> The 2008 Assessment also highlighted the role of detailed climate projections as requirements for some types of adaptation implementation. Useable and accessible data on future climate (temperature, precipitation) and sea level are often required by engineers and resource managers, for example, to determine timely, appropriate and cost-effective adaptation. For instance, data of past trends and future climate projections may be needed to inform decisions on upgrading and replacing infrastructure (such as pipelines, culverts and structures for shoreline protection), planning for hydroelectric facility placement and renovation, and selecting tree species for forestry operations. (p. 257)

In this instance, the term *accessible* directly relates to *access* of data by "engineers and resource managers, for example" (Eyzaguirre & Warren, 2014, p. 257), with no reference to the accessibility needs of persons with disabilities.

These findings were consistent across the data set, with coding across the documents linking the terms accessible/accessibility with matters unrelated to persons with disabilities. Another example is found in the report *Human Health in a Changing Climate: A Canadian Assessment of Vulnerabilities and Adaptive Capacity* (Seguin, 2008), a 484-page document. The terms *disabilities* and *persons with disabilities* are not found in this assessment. The term accessible is only found in three places in this report, within a similar context to the above extracts. In this assessment of *vulnerabilities* and *adaptive capacity*, speaking to the merits of adaptation to climate change, Seguin (2008) notes:

> Many adaptation options are accessible and affordable. For example, buildings can be protected from lightning at limited cost according to a National Standard of Canada for Lightning Protection Systems. (p. 94)

Relatedly, the term accessibility only appears once in this 484-page document, where Seguin (2008) speaks to food security in northern communities:

> Climate change and variability are influencing the distribution, availability and accessibility of wildlife that contributes to the diet of most Northerners. (p. 17)

These extracts further exemplify how across the data set, *accessible* and *accessibility* are never directly nor explicitly linked to persons with disabilities. Image descriptions and other options for making these reports more accessible to persons with disabilities are also not found. My findings indicate these public documents lack accessibility for many persons with disabilities in both their medium and their message.

The Contradictory Nature of the Data

Along with the mixed meanings associated with accessibility outlined above, I identified discrepancies between one or more government documents in my reflexive thematic analysis. That is, it became clear that the data sources were infused with contradictions. Once key example is where I have illustrated that adaptation in the government strategies is framed as an integral solution to climate change, while simultaneously the government presents research that fails to uphold adaptation to climate change as a successful approach. For instance, the Government of Canada (2016a) poster asks Canadians to adapt to climate change now, yet as mentioned earlier, in the *Human*

Health chapter by Berry, et al. (2014), the authors cite Lesnikowski et al. (2011) who found that information about climate change adaptation success is limited.

Another related example of contradictions is from Chapter 9 (Eyzaguirre & Warren, 2014), as the authors cite Ford et al. (2013) who state:

> A lack of consistent characterizations of adaptation – and specifically of 'successful' adaptation – are among the current challenges to monitoring and evaluating adaptation progress. (p. 261)

That is, embedded within hundreds of pages of government strategies pushing for climate change adaptation, is research that suggests it may not be a viable solution.

In the same chapter, I call attention to the last sentence of the corresponding eight lines that describe *the adaptation process* (Figure 4 above). Embedded within numerous pages suggesting that adaptation be employed through a specified process, Eyzaguirre and Warren (2014) provide an acknowledgement that "less progress is *evident* along the remaining three steps, although some examples of implementation of targeted actions are documented" (p. 260). That is, what is concealed within a vast array of adaptation-focused texts and figures is the fact that there are no confident measures or trusted evaluations of adaptation processes and adaptation outcomes. Returning to Figure 4, the admission that implementing targeted adaptation actions (phase 5); measuring and evaluating progress (phase 6); and learning, sharing knowledge and adjusting (phase 7) has not been achieved, may be the most relevant of all the adaptation research. That is, the government presents adaptation as a primary solution to effects of climate change while admitting that evidence does not exist for the efficacy of adaptation. Further, in the *Human Health in a Changing Climate: A Canadian Assessment of Vulnerabilities and Adaptive Capacity* (Seguin, 2008) report, the author states "There is a paucity of peer-reviewed studies on climate change and health adaptation and adaptive capacity in Canada" (p. 376). In other words, individuals are being asked to add more tasks (and in many cases more burdens) to their daily lives without substantial research confirming the usefulness of these adaptation efforts.

Incongruities and exclusions are further illustrated in Chapter 9, *Adaptation: Linking Research and Practice*, as it begins with Eyzaguirre and Warren (2014) stating that:

> Since 2008, climate change adaptation research and practice in Canada has been characterized by increasing engagement, diversity and complexity. Understanding of the adaptation process has improved, more groups are involved in adaptation discussions. (p. 255)

As demonstrated early in my findings, the document authors and contributors to these discussions are primarily government employees and environmental consultants. These select contributors cite increasing engagement and diversity, yet I did not find a single reference to consultation or collaboration with persons with disabilities. Contradictions are exemplified when increased engagement, diversity, and complexity in climate change research and practice is cited, while at the same time said persons and perspectives are excluded in these government publications.

Another example of the contradictory nature of the government documents occurs when the Canadian government asks individuals to take personal responsibility for adaptation, yet within the Berry et al. (2014) chapter, the authors cite the Canadian Medical Association's (2010) assertion that "successful adaptation requires inter-sectoral collaboration e.g., health, environment, planning, transport, infrastructure" (p. 217). These contradictions are interspersed throughout the documents and may lead to confusion for many individuals who are accessing these documents looking for tools to help themselves and others in a changing climate. Contradictions across the data set coalesce with themes of exclusion, individual responsibility, and assumptions of a normative body-mind. Given these findings, I consider the possibility that no matter how sophisticated we make our adaptation approaches, they may not ultimately succeed in protecting persons with disabilities in the face of climate change.

CHAPTER FIVE: Discussion

In this final chapter, I summarize my reflexive research method and findings, offer my interpretations and provocations, list implications, and conclude with my hope for more critical, thoughtful, and politicized climate change strategies.

Through a reflexive thematic data analysis, I sought to discover how health and disability were deployed in Canadian climate change documents. As such, my data was comprised of six Canadian climate change documents recommended to me by Canada's Minister of Environment and Climate Change in response to my query about relevant government strategies for persons with disabilities in the face of climatic threats. Since I was particularly curious about how disability was presented within the context of climate change research and strategies, a reflexive thematic analysis offered a path to investigate the data while keeping my own politics close at hand. When utilizing this type of qualitative research methodology, Braun and Clarke (2019) note that our own positions are always deeply embedded, and it is good practice to identify and reflect on what we assume and how these assumptions fit within our research findings. In turn, I have attempted to draw lines between my own politics and positioning and the conclusions I have derived from the data.

Reflexive Interpretations

As illustrated in my analysis, the Canadian Federal Government clearly prioritizes adaptation, resilience building, economics, and individualized climate mitigation efforts within the data. Goodley (2014) suggests that ableism clings to economic and ideological conditions. That is, in the documents I have seen what Goodley (2014) coined *neoliberal-ablism* – a system that values normal body-minds that are economically independent while still reliant on neoliberal capital production. Indeed, prioritization of the economy has historically infringed upon the rights of persons with disabilities and their ability to exercise autonomy and inclusion (Scanlon et al., 2014). As I have demonstrated, when barriers and challenges to climate change adaptation are presented, they do not include the unique needs of persons with disabilities. As such, I see these publications as ableist sites in which perspectives and knowledge held by persons with disabilities are missing, since a normalized body-mind is presented as the Canadian for whom these climate strategies are designed.

Through my disability justice politic, and specifically through a critical disability studies lens, I challenge the tacit assumption that adaptation is a one-size-fits-all approach to the threats of climate change. As I have shown, adaptation priorities are presented without consideration for the unique and varied needs of persons with disabilities. That is, an able-bodied, able-minded, and financially secure person is presumed in these suggestions when the authors make sweeping assumptions about adaptation means and capabilities. In addition to this presumption, I also found that these Federal Government climate change strategies capture important taken-for-granted notions about a uniform ability to adapt. For example, in the poster produced by the Government of Canada (2018), people who live in poverty, people experiencing homelessness, and the disabled are not considered. The dominant message presented in these publications is that government experts know best, and individual citizens are now responsible for themselves. Here, adaptation is framed as a necessary collective action, and Canadians are asked to individualize their responses to climate change and prepare for the ensuing threats through their own means. As a social worker, I see this individualized approach to climate change adaptation as problematic for those who rely on fixed monthly government assistance programs, for those who are isolated and/or immobile, and for those who are otherwise marginalized. In the individualized call to adapt to climate change, the government suggests Canadians take more adaptive action without providing more support to fulfill those proposed tasks.

The Cyclical Nature of Ableism

I connect the ableist notions I found in the climate change strategies with the broader societal ableism experienced by persons with disabilities. To help summarize my findings, I have designed a visual aid to illuminate the cyclical and exclusionary nature of ableism within these climate change documents and elsewhere. Goodley et al. (2018) suggest that it is not possible to separate the discursive from the material, since these conditions are intricately connected. The following figure visually conveys how ableism is perpetuated within Canadian climate change strategies and our material realities:

Figure 8

The Productive and Cyclical Nature of Ableism

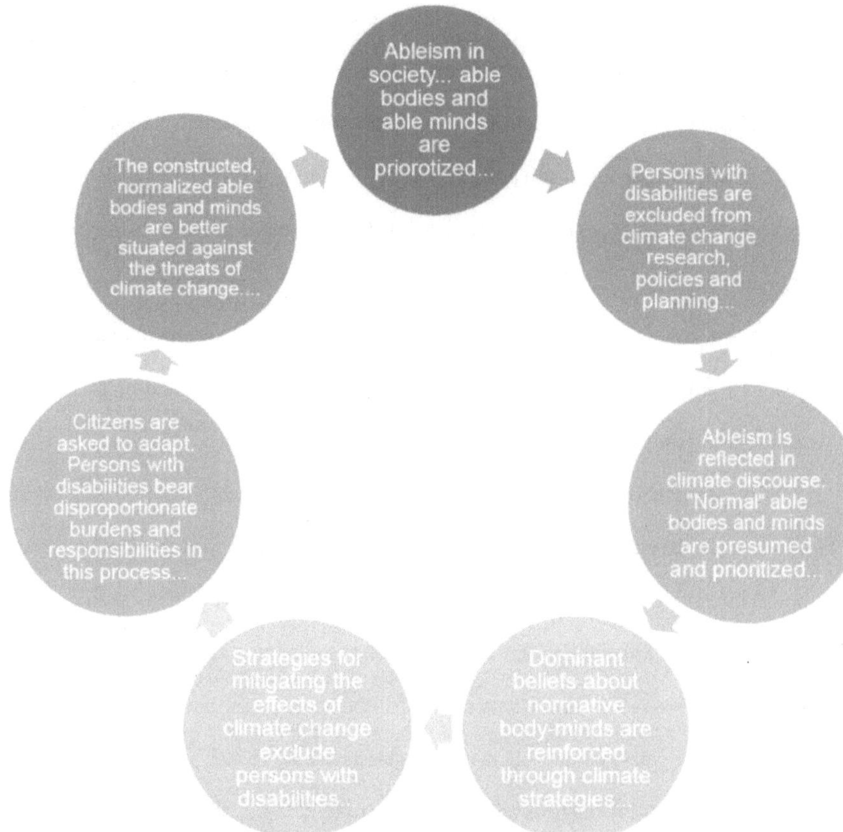

[IMAGE DESCRIPTION: A figure with eight shaded grey text circles linked by seven grey clockwise arrows with white text inside. Each circle depicts a facet of the cyclical nature of ableism in the context of both Canadian climate change publications and broader society.]

Note. The above diagram illustrates the productive and cyclical nature of ableism as manifested in Canadian climate change publications as well as in broader society.

Implications for Policy and Future Research

Through my critical analysis, and specifically within my findings, I have exposed ableist assumptions that shape Canadian climate change strategies. I have demonstrated that ableism is perpetuated through what is presented at face value as politically neutral territory. Taken-for-granted beliefs and assumptions about body-minds in the data are constantly shaping our social and political worlds. At the same time, I am challenged to uncover hegemonic notions of normal and valuable body-minds not only as they appear in the climate documents, but as they arise in my thinking, social work practice, and research. During the course of this study, for example, I have been pressed to consider such practical inclusions as image descriptions, and likewise, I call for greater consideration to accessibility in academia.

Not surprisingly, my data analysis revealed that persons with disabilities continue to be marginalized within the new terrain of government climate strategies and policies. With this injustice in mind, Goodley et al. (2018) note that critical disability studies positions disability as a political site around which to mobilize. As such, I utilized an intentionally reflexive analysis to help me contribute to a growing body of literature and activism that recognizes climate change strategies as deeply ableist, politicized, and partial. Relatedly, Belser (2020) suggests an allied resistance within social disability models and environmental justice by pointing to the political merits of moving from an individualized pathology to collective mobilizing. In essence, both disability justice and climate justice call us to see persons with disabilities as best positioned to understand their unique situations and to seek solutions to the challenges they face. I also advise caution, that the urgency of the changing climate does not grant permission to act unjustly in the name of its exigency.

If, as adaptation critiques suggest, the government's current approach proves unhelpful to *all* individuals who face climate change, then we are left with a society structured just as it is now. In this scenario, the elite, affluent, able-bodied, and able-minded are better situated to protect themselves from climatic threats and further harms. Without intersectional social justice perspectives taking a front seat in government climate policies, systemic inequities (such as ableism, classism, settler colonialism, and racism) will persist in climate-change planning.

Limitations

While reflecting on the limitations of this study, I return to my framework for anti-oppressive research, in which Strega (2015) asks social science researchers to gauge our helpfulness and political implications when using feminist poststructural research in marginalized communities. Specifically, Strega (2015, p. 145) provides three guideposts through which to evaluate feminist poststructural research: what is the political usefulness of our research; who benefits from our research; how reflexive we are with our complicity in the research. While I have attempted to answer these questions within the body of this thesis particularly through my reflexive disability justice politic, there are further points to consider.

It is important to note that this type of research tends to evade absolutes, as poststructuralism often begs more questions than gives clear answers. Marshall and Rossman (2015) point out that postmodern thinkers prefer methodologies that de-emphasize certainties of truth claims while leaving space for interpreting these truths. Similarly, throughout this research journey, and the complex terrains I contended with, I am left with more questions than answers. While I have included select perspectives, voices, bodies, and minds (from my own white, settler viewpoint), there are other meaningful experiences left out of my analysis. Specifically, I note that persons with disabilities do not constitute a homogenous group. That is, even if individuals identify as having (or have been diagnosed with) the same condition, their experiences and needs will often be intersectional and distinct. This reality underscores the need for more studies to represent the unique and varied experiences of disability within a changing climate, such as perspectives from BIPOC (Black, Indigenous, People of Colour) communities.

Indigenous Knowledge

Through a personal commitment to work anti-oppressively, I kept returning to relationships and meaningful conversations across these issues. Recently, I took part in Living Lands and Indigenous Climate Solutions: Responsibilities beyond Territorial Acknowledgements, a workshop with local Indigenous knowledge holders and the University of Victoria. I listened to living histories, stories of traditional land-use, and colonial (climate change) impacts on coastal peoples and ecosystems. I have come to view listening as a powerful act, capable of transforming relationships and guiding research in a good way. Although it was beyond the purview of this project, the absence of Canadian Indigenous knowledge and perspectives within in these documents was striking. Climate change observations and initiatives from Indigenous communities were lacking in the documents, which pointed to a prioritization of select Canadians. When speaking about Indigenous peoples in Canada, the publications did not reference harms from colonial histories nor ongoing colonizing policies and practices. First People's voices were largely absent from government adaptation strategies (with no mention of people who identify both as Indigenous and as persons with disabilities). In the government documents,

Indigenous communities were often synonymous with northern communities, with the latter descriptor generally used to cite climate challenges for people in northern Canada, without naming colonization. Traditional Ecological Knowledge (TEK) was not given adequate consideration in the development of these documents and strategies. In fact, climate change threats to Indigenous communities were scarcely mentioned, and when challenges were included, they were presented as internal vulnerabilities posed as politically neutral zones. For example, in Chapter 7 of *Human Health*, low education levels were listed by Berry et al. (2014) as one adaptive capacity challenge; that is, a lack of colonial knowledge and education was cited as one reason young Indigenous people have reduced adaptive capacities. Reference to historical and current tensions between Indigenous communities and the Canadian government in areas such as land sovereignty, resource extraction, and reconciliation, were markedly missing from the publications. While government strategies quietly cite limits related to adaptation, they simultaneously present Indigenous communities as having several challenges adapting to climate change. The bitter irony of listing one climate challenge as Indigenous youth's failure to adopt a contemporary, colonial education is not lost here. At the same time, many scholars and Indigenous leaders have tied climate change to greenhouse gas emissions and other colonial processes (Cameron, 2012). Indeed, colonialism and capitalism were latent themes throughout the climate change documents I reviewed, yet these systems were not addressed by the government publications. For example, the data set referenced unequal access to resources and inter-jurisdictional issues as barriers to climate change adaptation in Aboriginal health systems (Berry et. al., 2014). Moreover, the authors do not adequately speak to the systemic barriers faced by Indigenous peoples; that is, they cite unequal access to resources without considering colonial systems of governance that constrain access to such resources. While it was beyond the capacity of this study to explore these findings with the care that they deserve, I point to the need for settler scientists and researchers to take seriously colonial legacies perpetuated in climate change strategies and policies. Reflecting on Canada's need for reconciliation in these matters, Steinstra (2015) states: "With the persistent involvement of Indigenous nations, women and others who resist, alternatives are imagined and created" (p. 647). These are complex problems with contentious histories and excluding these perspectives from research is an acknowledged limitation of the current study and the documents analyzed. Any socially just strategy (including climate justice pursuits) must create opportunities to further aid reconciliation and collaboration with Indigenous communities.

Future Directions for Climate Justice Research

Given the methods chosen and the scale of this project, additional limitations include making assumptions about the experiences of others — namely persons with disabilities, climate scientists, government employees, and contributors to these strategies. I am not so naïve as to postulate that the authors of and contributors to the data set are immune to health challenges and disabilities; rather, I see capitalism and neoliberalism as contributors to the stigmatization of illness and disability in politicized spaces, where maintaining the appearance of normal bestows authority, power, and wealth. As Van Aswegen and Shevlin (2019) note, "ableism, it is argued, has come to dominate the framework of thinking of society as a while, operating as a discourse of power and authority" (p. 636). Through constructing more critical and inclusive research projects, we are better able to reflect the heterogeneous nature of health and disability, including how ableism manifests within Canadian and global climate change initiatives. Comparing and contrasting similar mechanisms within international scholarship is another prudent pursuit, since these processes could elucidate context-specific human needs and limits to climate change and adaptation.

I suggest further research that judiciously analyzes resilience thinking in the context of adaptation to climate change is warranted. Similarly, within the context of climate resilience, Mikulewicz (2019) has questioned whether problems of inequity lie in resilience theories themselves, or whether governing bodies use the notion of resilience to propel neoliberal systems. Compared to relational theories of disability, resilience can be viewed as interactive, that is, increasing resilience for certain people may mean reducing resilience for others (Mikulewicz, 2019). I had hoped to find more studies that situate disability within climate science, as well as work that critically engages adaptation and resilience thinking. Still, I am encouraged to see these areas of scholarship growing, and I anticipate more issues of social justice will be brought to the fore of climate studies and climate policies.

While paying attention to possible versions of reality created through these climate change documents, I know that there are many truths that have been left out. I understand that my experiences of health and my climate change needs are not universal, and that I have not covered all of the unique perspectives of persons with disabilities. With this complexity in mind, I contemplate the similarities between those with invisible illnesses, and the ways in which many environmental and climate harms are unseen and therefore undetectable to those who have not experienced them. Certainly, this reality presents further challenges to mobilizing support for climate impacts on invisible illness and having governments take seriously the needs of people who exist out of sight. Indeed, the work of making these injustices visible is a heavy labour that falls on those who are already oppressed and often expended.

I have discovered much through this thesis journey and, as people began to share their stories with me, I included elements of this learning (such as image descriptions) in my work. Many persons with disabilities have reported that, even within grassroots and activist communities, many hold a "greener than thou" attitude (Fenney, 2017, p. 515). It is my hope that this study not only contributes to emancipatory and inclusive dialogues and practices in my life, but that it may touch the grassroots and academic fields of social work, climate justice, and disability justice in productive ways. Assuredly, I contend that ableism is not limited to government adaptation strategies; rather, it pervades many areas of society. I call for more scholarly engagement with the politics of critical disability studies and intersectionality within and across all domains.

The Elsewhen

Over the course of writing this thesis, there were many times that I felt dreadfully pessimistic about the future of our climate and the protection of persons with disabilities. It is clear to me that government climate change strategies stem from oppressive ideologies, which are propelled by forces such as ongoing settler colonialism, neoliberalism, capitalism, racism, sexism, and ableism. Although the unjust implications of these systems are far-reaching, they are not as sweeping and pervasive as I once believed. When I yearn for hope, I see countless places and spaces of resistance, of flourishing, and survival. Last year, I was heartened to watch thousands of citizens march on parliament (in Victoria and across the world) to protest not only climate change and ecological crises, but also in resistance to overlapping forces of injustice. These issues are no longer seen as singular and courageous individuals and communities are working to confront climate injustices and intersecting sites of marginalization.

When I look for them, I find many stories of resistance. For example, teenage activist and water protector Autumn Peltier, from the Wiikwemkoong First Nation on Manitoulin Island in Northern Ontario, is engaged in the fight to protect Indigenous water. Similarly, Quannah Chasinghorse, from the Han Gwich'in and Lakota Sioux Nations in Alaska, is helping to protect Artic wildlife and preserve well-being in her community in the face of climate change. Daphne Frias, a climate activist with physical disabilities from West Harlem, is addressing environmental racism in her New York neighbourhood. Additionally, teenage climate activist Great Thunberg is helping to lead millions toward a more just future internationally. As someone who identifies as being on the autism spectrum (as well as self-identifying with other health conditions), Thunberg openly claims her diagnosis as a superpower. In a similar testament to the natural marriage of these issues, Belser (2020) notes:

> Climate change asks us to grapple with loss, with change, with uncertainty, with fear. This is affective terrain that many disabled people know intimately. Might disability experience offer some meaningful strategies for reckoning with the embodied knowledge of human vulnerability, for gentling the dread this knowledge provokes, and for exploring the possibilities it opens? (para. 35)

Indeed, persons with disabilities often work creatively and persistently to tackle complex challenges related to survival. Who better to resource when planning for the inevitable hazards of climate change than communities who continuously resist the threat of extinction?

Situating a just future in the context of social work theory and practice is no different; that is, persons with disabilities are naturally in every community and must be an integral part of social justice and climate justice efforts. From an intersectional perspective, persons with disabilities have historically contended with tremendous loss and trauma, and social workers would do well to amplify these perspectives and experiences in all aspects of our work. By specifically questioning the limits to, and efficacy of, adapting to climate change, social workers can both protect themselves and their disabled clients by resisting the unwarranted harms and burdens placed on vulnerable populations. At the same time, through critical interrogations of what makes certain people and groups more vulnerable to diverse threats, social workers can expose the structural inequities and deep-seated roots of ableism within our society, our profession, and ourselves. Similarly, while building climate resilience may be a worthy endeavour, social workers committed to anti-oppressive practices must also challenge and question any system that requires vulnerable populations to carry more responsibility. That is, for resilience building to become a critical directive for persons with disabilities, there must be conditions and systems that actively threaten their well-being. Social work and social workers have important roles to play in challenging unjust social and climate policies, and we must bring attention to the many ways in which these systems already adversely impact persons with disabilities.

Finally, archaeologist and wilderness survivalist Chris Begley (2019), who studies collapsed societies, offers insights for surviving climate catastrophes; that is, Begley suggests that despite climate disasters, billions of people will remain entrenched in the messiness of society. We will still need to fix our broken systems. Kindness, courage, cooperation, and empathy are just as important as any survival skill, and, while our needs are immense, we must turn toward our problems, not away (Begley, 2019). My anti-oppressive work in this thesis comes on the heels of hundreds of years of survival and resistance from disabled people of colour and other historically marginalized communities. It remains that we cannot ignore injustice in pursuit of a better future since "no tragic yet convenient event will allow us to discard our complex, messy, and ever-changing social reality and live out our rugged, individualistic fantasy" (Begley, 2019).

Since we share this planet and its resources, embracing the complexity and fragility of life is crucial to moving toward a just future. In my opening epigraph, I quoted Alison Kafer (2013), who refers to an elsewhen in which disability is seen as vital, integral, and valuable. Akin to Kafer, I plead for further research and activism to move forward with the indispensable and intersectional knowledge offered by persons with disabilities, since this will advance understandings related to the challenges of climate change and the limits of adaptation for all people. This is my elsewhen.

What's Next

I am eager to share my finished thesis and auxiliary findings with others in my academic and social circles – communities that naturally include persons with disabilities. I anticipate hosting an accessible, virtual talk related to my research with invitations extended to the *Society of Students with Disabilities* at the University of Victoria. Our community often talks about how disability perspectives are essential when planning socially just initiatives as well as how we can best facilitate inclusion and equity. We understand interdependence is a critical part of our survival, and, as a community we endeavour to create spaces where disability is not a marginalized experience, where no body or mind is left behind. In closing, I also intend to share the findings of this thesis with the Canadian Federal Government, and I look forward to more conversations that centre persons with disabilities within Canadian climate change planning.

References

Alaimo, S. (2017). Foreword. In S. Jaquette Ray, & J. Sibara (Eds.), *Disability studies and the environmental humanities: Toward an eco-crip theory* (pp. ix-iv). University of Nebraska Press.

Adger, N.W., Dessai, S., Goulden, M., Hulme, M., Lorenzoni, I., Nelson, D.R., Naess, L.O., Wolf, J., & Wreford, A. (2009). Are there social limits to adaptation to climate change? *Climatic Change, 93*(3), 335-354. https://doi.org/10.1007/s10584-008-9520-z

Alam, G.M., Alam, K., & Mushtaq, S. (2017). Climate change perceptions and local adaptation strategies of hazard-prone rural households in Bangladesh. *Climate Risk Management, 17*, 52-63. https://doi.org/10.1016/j.crm.2017.06.006

Alston, M., & Whittenbury, K. (2010). *Research, action and policy: Addressing the gendered impacts of climate change*. Springer.

Alston, M. (2011) Gender and climate change in Australia. *Journal of Sociology, 47*(1), 53–70. https://doi.org/10.1177/1440783310376848

Alston, M. (2015). Social work, climate change and global cooperation. *International Social Work, 58*(3), 355-363. https://doi.org/10.1177/0020872814556824

Baker, J. (Ed.) (2012). *Climate change, disaster risk, and the urban poor: Cities building resilience for a changing world*. Urban Development. World Bank. https://doi.org/10.1596/978-0-8213-8845-7

Begley, C. (2019, September 23). *I study collapsed civilizations. Here's my advice for a climate change apocalypse*. Lexington Herald Leader. https://www.kentucky.com/opinion/op-ed/article235384162.html

Belser, J.W. (2020). Disability, Climate Change, and Environmental Violence: The Politics of Invisibility and the Horizon of Hope. *Disability Studies Quarterly*, *40*(4). https://doi.org/10.18061/dsq.v40i4.6959

Berry, H.L., Kelly, B.J., Hanigan, I.C., Coates, J.H., McMichael, A.J., Welsh, J.A., & Kjellstrom, T. (2008). *Rural mental health impacts of climate change*. The Australian National University.

Berry, P., Clarke, K., Fleury, M.D., & Parker, S. (2014). Human health. In F.J Warren & D.S. Lemmen (Eds.), *Canada in a changing climate: Sector perspectives on impacts and adaptation* (pp. 191-232). Government of Canada.

Braun, V., & Wilkinson, S. (2003). Liability or asset? Women talk about the vagina. *Psychology of Women Section Review*, *5*(2), 28-42. https://doi.org/10.3138/cjhs.262-a3

Braun, V., & Clarke, V. (2006). Using thematic analysis in psychology. *Qualitative Research in Psychology, 3*(2), 77-101. https://doi.org/10.1191/1478088706qp063oa

Braun, V., & Clarke, V. (2017). Thematic analysis. *The Journal of Positive Psychology, 12*(3), 297-298. https://doi.org/10.1080/17439760.2016.1262613

Braun, V., & Clarke, V. (2018). Using thematic analysis in counselling and psychotherapy research: A critical reflection. *Counselling and Psychotherapy Research, 18(*2). https://doi.org/10.1002/capr.12165

Braun, V., & Clarke, V. (2019). Reflecting on reflexive thematic analysis. *Qualitative Research in Sport, Exercise, and Health, 11*(4), 589-597. https://doi.org/10.1080/2159676X.2019.1628806

Braun, V., & Clarke, V., Hayfield, N. (2019). A starting point for your journey, not a map: Nikki Hayfield in conversation with Virginia Braun and Victoria Clarke about thematic analysis. *Qualitative Research in Psychology.* https://doi.org/10.1080/14780887.2019.1670765

Braun, V., & Clarke, V. (2020). One size fits all? What counts as quality practice in (reflexive) thematic analysis. *Qualitative Research in Psychology.* https://doi.org/10.1080/14780887.2020.1769238

Brodie, J. (2007). Reforming social justice in neoliberal times. *Studies in Social Justice, 1*(2), 93-107. https://doi.org/10.26522/ssj.v1i2.972

Brooks, N., Adger, W.N., & Kelly, P.M. (2005). The determinants of vulnerability and adaptive capacity at the national level and the implications for adaptation. *Global Environmental Climate Change, 15*(2), 151-163. https://doi.org/10.1016/j.gloenvcha.2004.12.006

Bush, E., Lemmen, D.S. (2019). *Canada's Changing Climate Report.* Government of Canada. https://changingclimate.ca/CCCR2019/

Butler, J. (2016, March 30). *Why preserve the life of the other? Tanner lectures on human values – interpreting non-violence* [Video]. YouTube. https://www.youtube.com/watch?v=40YPnzv5JzM

Cameron, E.S. (2012). Securing Indigenous politics: A critique of the vulnerability and adaptation approach to the human dimensions of climate change in the Canadian Arctic. *Global Environmental Change, 22*(1), 103-114. https://doi.org/10.1016/j.gloenvcha.2011.11.004

Canadian Medical Association. (2010). *National health goals for Canada: A review of successes, challenges, and opportunities for the Canadian Medical Association.*

Campbell, F.K. (2009). *Contours of ableism: Territories, objects, disability and desire*. Palgrave Macmillan.

Caria, S., Hayes, A. (2019, September 24). *The problem with the phrase 'and other vulnerable groups'*. Devex. https://www.devex.com/news/sponsored/opinion-the-problem-with-the-phrase-and-other-vulnerable-groups-94543

Clare, E. (2017). Notes on natural worlds, disabled bodies and a politics of cure. In S. Jaquette Ray, & J. Sibara (Eds.), *Disability studies and the environmental humanities* (pp. 242-265). University of Nebraska Press.

Clayton, S. Manning, C., Krygsman, K., & Speiser, M. (2017). *Mental health and our changing climate: Impacts, implications, and guidance*. American Psychological Association & ecoAmerica. https://www.apa.org/news/press/releases/2017/03/mental-health-climate.pdf

Crenshaw, K. (1989). Demarginalizing the intersection of race and sex: A black feminist critique of antidiscrimination doctrine, feminist theory, and antiracist politics. *University of Chicago Legal Forum, 1*, 139-167.

Crenshaw, K. (1991). Mapping the margins: Intersectionality, identity politics, and violence against women of color. *Stanford Law Review, 43*(6), 1241-1299.

Crow, C. (1996). Including all of our lives. In J Morris (Eds.), *Encounters with strangers* (pp.1-21). The Women's Press Ltd.

Cumby, T. (2016). *Climate change and social work: Our roles and barriers to action* (1828) [Master's Thesis, Wilfred Laurier University]. Theses and Dissertations Comprehensive. https://scholars.wlu.ca/etd/1828

Czyzewski, K., Tester, F. (2014). Social work, colonial history and engaging Indigenous self-determination. *Canadian Social Work Review*, 31(2), 211-226. http://www.jstor.org/stable/43486322

Dankelman, I. (Ed.). (2010). *Gender and Climate Change: An Introduction* (1st ed.). Routledge.

Davis, L. (2013). *The End of Normal: Identity in a Biocultural Era*. University of Michigan Press.

Diamond, I., & Quinby, L. (1988). *Feminism & Foucault: Reflections on resistance.* Northeastern University Press.

Dingo, R. (2007). Making the "unfit, fit": The rhetoric of mainstreaming in the World Bank's commitment to gender equality and disability rights. *Wagadu, 4*(Summer), 93-107.

http://sites.cortland.edu/wagadu/wp-content/uploads/sites/3/2014/02/dingo.pdf

Dominelli, L. (2018). *The Routledge Handbook of Green Social Work*. London, Routledge.

Ekers, M., Hart, G., Kipfer, S., & Loftus, A. (2012). *Gramsci: Space, Nature, Politics*. John Wiley & Sons Incorporated.

Erickson, C. (2018). *Environmental Justice as Social Work Practice*. Oxford University Press.

Eyzaguirre, J., & Warren, F.J. (2014). Adaptation: Linking research and practice. In F.J. Warren & D.S. Lemmen (Eds.), *Canada in a changing climate: Sector perspectives on impacts and adaptation* (pp. 253-286). Government of Canada.

Fayerman, P., & Mahichi, B. (2018, August 18). B.C. wildfires 2018: Medical issues surge as air quality advisory becomes longest on record. *Vancouver Sun*. https://vancouversun.com/news/local-news/wildfires-2018-medical-issues-surge-as-air-quality-advisory-becomes-longest-on-record

Fenney, D. (2017). Ableism and disablism in the UK environmental movement. *Environmental Values, 26*(4), 503-522. https://doi.org/10.3197/096327117X14976900137377

Filho W.L., & Nalau J (Eds.). (2018) *Limits to climate change adaptation*. Springer. https://doi.org/10.1007/978-3-319-64599-5

Filho W.L, & Knieling, J. (Eds.). (2013). *Climate Change Governance*. Springer eBooks. https://doi.org/10.1007/978-3-642-29831-8

Fleming, A., Michaelson, R., Youssef, A., & Holmes, O. (2018, August 13). Heat: The next big inequality issue. *The Guardian*. https://www.theguardian.com/cities/2018/aug/13/heat-next-big-inequality-issue-heatwaves-world

Foucault, M. (2003). Society must be defended [Lecture series at the Collège de France] (D. Macey, Trans.) Paris, France: Collège de France (Original lectures 1975-1976).

Foucault, M. (1980). *Power/knowledge: Selected interviews and other writings 1972-1977*. C. Gordon (Ed.). Harvester.

Foucault, M. (1986). Of other spaces. *Diacritics, 16*(1), 22-27.

Fritsch, K. (2017). Toxic pregnancies: Speculative futures, disabling environments, and neoliberal biocapital. In S. Jaquette Ray, & J. Sibara (Eds.), *Disability studies and the environmental humanities* (pp. 359-380). University of Nebraska Press.

Gaard, G. (2015). Ecofeminism and climate change. *Women's Studies International Forum, 49*, 20-33. https://doi.org/10.1016/j.wsif.2015.02.004

Gifford, R. (2011). The dragons of inaction: Psychological barriers that limit climate change mitigation and adaptation. *The American Psychologist, 66*(4), 290-302. https://doi.org/10.1037/a0023566

Garland-Thomson, R. (2005). Feminist disability studies. *Signs: Journal of Women in Culture and Society, 30*(2), 1557-1587. https://doi.org/10.1086/423352

Gaskin, C., Taylor, D., Kinnear, S., Mann, J., Hillman, W., & Moran, M. (2017). Factors associated with the climate change vulnerability and the adaptive capacity of people with disability: A systematic review. *American Meteorological Society, 9*(4), 801-814. https://doi.org/10.1175/WCAS-D-16-0126.1

Goodley, D. (2014). *Dis/ability studies: Theorising disablism and ableism.* Routledge.

Goodley, D. 2016. *Disability Studies: An Interdisciplinary Introduction* (2nd ed.). Sage.

Goodley,D., Liddiard, K., & Runswick-Cole, K. (2018). Feeling disability: theories of affect and critical disability studies. *Disability & Society, 33*(2), 197-217. https://doi.org/10.1080/09687599.2017.1402752

Goodley, D., & Lawthom, R. (2019). Critical disability studies, Brexit and Trump: a time of neoliberal–ableism. *Rethinking History, 23*(2), 233-251. https://doi.org/10.1080/13642529.2019.1607476

Government of Canada. (2016a). *Adapting to our Changing Climate in Canada.* [Poster presentation]. https://www.nrcan.gc.ca/sites/www.nrcan.gc.ca/files/earthsciences/images/asses s/2016/adaptation_poster_e.jpg

Government of Canada. (2016b). *Working Group on Adaptation and Climate Resilience.* https://www.canada.ca/content/dam/eccc/migration/cc/content/6/4/7/64778dd 5-e2d9-4930-be59-d6db7db5cbc0/wg_report_acr_e_v5.pdf

Grue, J. (2011). Discourse analysis and disability: some topics and issues. *Disability and Society, 22*(5), 532-546. https://doi.org/10.1177/0957926511405572

Hall, K. Q. (2017). Cripping sustainability, realizing food justice. In S. Jaquette Ray, & J. Sibara (Eds.), *Disability studies and the environmental humanities: Toward an eco-crip theory* (pp. 422-446). University of Nebraska Press.

Hammerlsy, M. (2003). Conversation analysis and discourse analysis: Methods or paradigms? *Discourse and Society, 14*(6), 751-781. https://doi.org/10.1177/09579265030146004

Henly-Shepard, S. (2018). Resilience in Action: Climate & Ecosystem-Inclusive Disaster Risk Reduction. Mercy Corps. https://resiliencelinks.org/system/files/documents/2019-08/real_ria_climate_final_mar_2019508_0.pdf

Henriques, J., Hollway, W., Urwin, C., Venn, C., & Walkerdine, V. (1984). *Changing the subject: Psychology, social regulation, and subjectivity*. Routledge.

International Energy Agency. (2018). *World Energy Outlook*. Paris. https://www.iea.org/reports/world-energy-outlook-2018

IPCC. (2007). *Climate Change 2007: Synthesis Report. Contribution of Working Groups I, II and III to the Fourth Assessment Report of the Intergovernmental Panel on Climate Change.* https://www.ipcc.ch/site/assets/uploads/2018/02/ar4_syr_full_report.pdf

IPCC. (2012). *Managing the Risks of Events and Disasters to Advance Climate Change Adaptation.* https://www.ipcc.ch/site/assets/uploads/2018/03/SREX_Full_Report-1.pdf

IPCC. (2014). *Climate change 2014: Impacts, adaptation, and vulnerability.* https://www.ipcc.ch/report/ar5/wg2/

IPCC. (2018). *Global Warming of 1.5°C. An IPCC Special Report on the impacts of global warming of 1.5°C above pre-industrial levels and related global greenhouse gas emission pathways, in the context of strengthening the global response to the threat of climate change, sustainable development, and efforts to eradicate poverty*. https://www.ipcc.ch/sr15/

Israel, A.L., & Sachs, C. (2012). A Climate for feminist intervention: Feminist science studies and climate change. In M. Alston & K. Whittenbury (Eds.)., *Research action and policy: Addressing the gendered impacts of climate change*. Springer. https://doi.org/10.1007/978-94-007-5518-5

Jodoin, S., Ananthamoorthy, N., & Lofts, K. (2020). A Disability Rights Approach to Climate Governance. *Ecology Law Quarterly*, *47*(1), 73-116. https://doi.org/10.2139/ssrn.3610193

Jóhannesson, I. Á. 2010. The Politics of Historical Discourse Analysis: A Qualitative Research Method? *Discourse: Studies in the Cultural Politics of Education*, *31*(2), 251–264. https://doi.org/10.1080/01596301003679768

Johnson, V.A. (2017). Bringing together feminist disability studies and environmental justice. In S. Jaquette Ray, & J. Sibara (Eds.), *Disability studies and the environmental humanities: Toward an eco-crip theory* (pp. 73-93). University of Nebraska Press.

Kafer, A. (2013). *Feminist, queer, crip*. Indianapolis: Indiana University Press.

Kafer, A. (2017, April 6). Health rebels: A crip manifesto for social justice [Video]. YouTube. https://www.youtube.com/watch?v=YqcOUD1pBKw

Kosanic, A., Petzold, J., Dunham, A., & Razanajatovo, M. (2019). Climate concerns and the disabled community. *Science, 366*(6466), 698-699. https://doi.org/10.1126/science.aaz9045

Lesnikowski, A.C., Ford, J.D., Berrang-Ford, L., Paterson, J.A., Barrera, M., & Heymann, S.J. (2011). Adapting to health impacts of climate change: A study of UNFCCC Annex I parties. *Environmental Research Letters*, *6*(4), 1-9. https://doi.org/10.1088/1748-9326/6/4/044009

Macgregor, S. (2014). Only Resist: Feminist Ecological Citizenship and the Post-politics of Climate Change. *Hypatia,* 29(3), 617-633.

Malhotra, R., & Isitt, B. (2017). *Disabling barriers: Social movements, disability history, and the law*. UBC Press.

Marshall, C., & Rossman, G.B. (2015). *Designing qualitative research*. SAGE Publications.

McCruer, R. (2006). *Crip theory: Cultural signs of queerness and disability*. Temple University Press.

Melograna, J. (Director). (2015). *The Right to be Rescued* [Film]. Rooted in Rights.

Metzl, J.M., & Kirkland, A. (2010). *Against health: How health became the new morality*. New York University Press.

Mingus, M. (2011, February 12). Changing the Framework: Disability Justice. How our communities can move beyond access to wholeness [Blog Post]. https://leavingevidence.wordpress.com/2011/02/12/changing-the-framework-disability-justice/

Moosa-Mitha, M. (2015). Situating anti-oppressive theories within critical and difference centred perspectives. In L. Brown, & S. Strega (2nd Eds.), *Research as resistance: Revisiting critical, Indigenous and anti-oppressive approaches* (pp. 37-72). Toronto: Canadian Scholars Press/Women's Press.

Nocella II, A.J. (2017). Defining eco-ability: Social justice and the intersectionality of disability, nonhuman animals, and ecology. In S. Jaquette Ray, & J. Sibara (Eds.), *Disability studies and the environmental humanities: Toward an eco-crip theory* (pp. 141-167). University of Nebraska Press.

Noelke, C., McGovern, M, Corsi, D.J., Jimenez, M.P., Stern, I.A., Wing, S., Berkman, L. (2016). Increasing ambient temperature reduces emotional well-being. *Environmental Research, 151*, 124-129. https://doi.org/10.1016/j.envres.2016.06.045

Oksala, J. (2018). Feminism, capitalism and ecology. *Hypatia: A Journal of Feminist Philosophy, 33*(2), 216-234. https://doi.org/10.1111/hypa.12395

Park, Y., Crath, R., Jeffery, D. (2018). Disciplining the risky subject: a discourse analysis of the concept of resilience in social work literature. *Journal of Social Work, 20*(2), 152-172. https://10.1177/1468017318792953

Pon, G. (2009). Cultural competency as new racism: An ontology of forgetting. *Journal of Progressive Human Services, 20*(1), 59-71. https://doi.org/10.1080/10428230902871173

Ribot, J. (2011). Vulnerability before adaptation: Toward transformative climate action. *Global Environmental* Change, *21*(4), 1160-1162. https://doi.org/10.1016/j.gloenvcha.2011.07.008

Rimmerman, A. (2013). *Social Inclusion of People with Disabilities: National and International Perspectives.* Cambridge University Press.

Rose, N. (1999). *Powers of freedom. Reframing political thought.* Cambridge: Cambridge University Press.

Saito, O., Kranjac-Berisavljevic, G., Takeuchi, K., & Gyasi, E.A. (2018). *Strategies for building resilience against climate and ecosystem changes in Sub-Saharan Africa*. Springer Nature Singapore.

Santamouris, M. (2019). *Minimizing energy consumption, energy poverty and global and local climate change in the built environment: Innovating to zero*. Elsevier Inc.

Schirato, T., Danaher, G., Webb, J. (2012). *Understanding Foucault: A Critical Introduction*. London: Routledge.

Seguin, J. (2008). *Human health in a changing climate: a Canadian assessment of vulnerabilities and adaptive capacity: Synthesis report*. Health Canada. https://publications.gc.ca/site/eng/9.691579/publication.html

Shindell, D., Zhang, Y., Scott, M., Ru, M., Stark, K., & Ebi, K.L. (2020). The effects of heat exposure on human mortality throughout the United States. *GeoHealth*, *4*(4), 1-12. https://doi.org/10.1029/2019GH000234

Shakespeare, T., & Watson, N. (2010). Beyond models: Understanding the complexity of disabled people's lives. In G. Scambler & S. Scambler (Eds.), *New directions in the sociology of chronic and disabling conditions: Assaults on the lifeworld.* Palgrave Macmillan.

Simpson, N. (2017). Disabling justice? The exclusion of people with disabilities from the food justice movement. In S. Jaquette Ray, & J. Sibara (Eds.), *Disability studies and the environmental humanities* (pp. 402-421). University of Nebraska Press.

St. Pierre, J. (2017). Becoming Dysfluent: Fluency as Biopolitics and Hegemony. *Journal of Literary & Cultural Disability Studies, 11*(3), 339-356.

Statistics Canada. (2016, February 29). *Canadian survey on disability 2012: Data tables.* https://www150.statcan.gc.ca/n1/pub/89-654-x/89-654-x2016001-eng.htm

Stienstra, D. (2015). Northern Crises. *International Feminist Journal of Politics, 17*(4), 630-651. https://doi.org/10.1080/14616742.2015.1060695

Strega, S. (2015). The view from the poststructural margins: Epistemology and methodology reconsidered. In L. Brown, & S. Strega (2nd Eds.), *Research as resistance: Revisiting critical, Indigenous and anti-oppressive approaches* (pp. 119-152). Toronto: Canadian Scholars Press/Women's Press.

Tschakert, P. (2007). Views from the vulnerable: Understanding climatic and other stressors in the Sahel. *Global Environmental Change, 17*(3–4), 381-396. https://doi.org/10.1016/j.gloenvcha.2006.11.008

Thiesmeyer, L. (2003). *Discourse and silencing.* John Benjamins Publishing Company.

Thomas, C., (2007). *Sociologies of disability and illness: Contested ideas in disability studies and medical Sociology*. Palgrave Macmillian.

Van Aswegen, J., Shevlin, M. (2019). *Disabling Discourses and Ableist Assumptions: Reimaging social justice through education for disabled people through a critical discourse analysis approach. Policy Futures in Education, 17*(5), 635-656. https://doi.org/10.1177/1478210318817420

Wakefield, A., & Fleming, J. (2009). *The SAGE dictionary of policing*. SAGE Publications.

Walker, R., Mason, W. (2015). *Climate Change Adaptation for Health and Social Services*. CSIRO Publishing.

Warren, F.J., & Lemmen, D.S. (2014). *Canada in a changing climate: Sector perspectives on impacts and adaptation*. Government of Canada. https://www.nrcan.gc.ca/climate-change/impacts-adaptations/canada-changing-climate-sector-perspectives-impacts-and-adaptation/16309

Webb, M. (2011). On confluences and divergences. *Dialogues in Human Geography, 1*(1), 84-89.

Weissbecker, I. (2011). *Climate Change and Human Well-Being: Global Challenges and Opportunities*. New York, NY: Springer.

Wheeler, T., & von Braun, J. (2013). Climate change impacts on global food security. *Science, 341*(6145), 508-513. https://doi.org/10.1126/science.1239402

Willig, C. (2013). *Introducing qualitative research in psychology* (3rd ed.). Open University Press.

Withers, A.J. (2012). *Disability politics & theory*. Fernwood Publishing Company.

Wolbring, G. (2008). The Politics of Ableism. *Development, 51*(2), 252-258. https://doi.org/10.1057/dev.2008.17

Wolbring, G. (2009). A culture of neglect: Climate discourse and disabled people. *M/C Journal, 12*(4). https://doi.org/10.5204/mcj.173

Wolbring, G., & Leopatra, V. (2012). Climate Change, Water, Sanitation and Energy Insecurity: Invisibility of People with Disabilities. *Canadian Journal of Disability Studies, 1*(3), 66–90. https://doi.org/10.15353/cjds.v1i3.58

World Health Organization. (2011). *World report on disability*. https://www.who.int/disabilities/world_report/2011/report.pdf

www.ingramcontent.com/pod-product-compliance
Lightning Source LLC
LaVergne TN
LVHW041102150826
845673LV00007B/1887

* 9 7 8 3 3 8 4 2 8 0 2 5 1 *